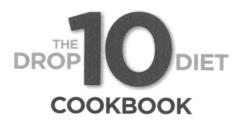

THE DROP 10 DIET COOKBOOK

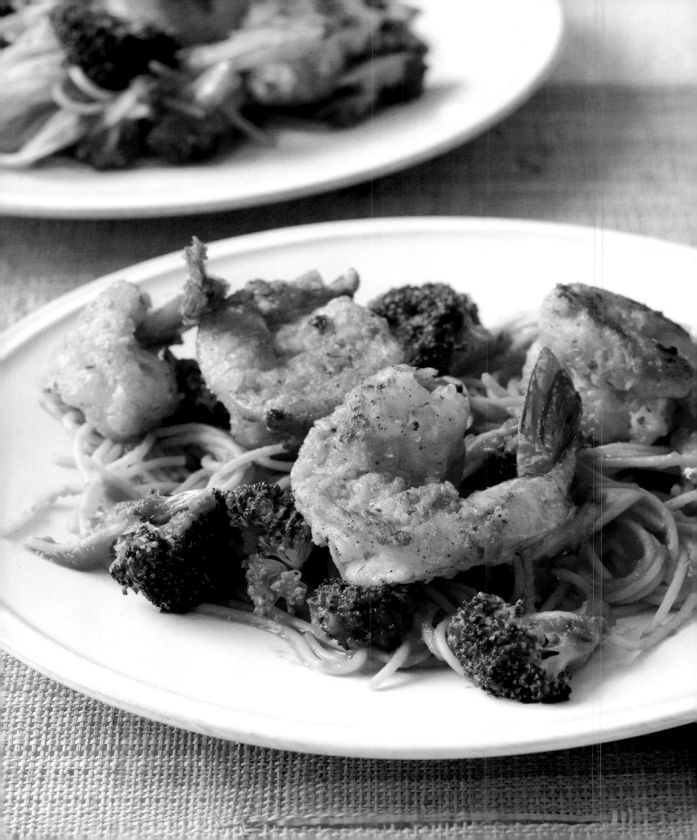

THE DROP 10 DIET COOKBOOK

More Than 100 Tasty, Easy Superfood
Recipes That Effortlessly Peel Off Pounds

LUCY DANZIGER

Beth Janes and the Editors of *SELF* Magazine

BALLANTINE BOOKS | NEW YORK

LIBRARY OF CONGRESS CATALOGING-IN-PUBLICATION DATA
Danziger, Lucy S.
The drop 10 diet cookbook : more than 100 tasty, easy superfood
recipes that effortlessly peel off pounds /
Lucy Danziger, editor in chief, *SELF* magazine.
pages cm
Includes index.
ISBN 978-0-345-53166-7 (pbk.) — ISBN 978-0-345-53168-1 (ebook)
1. Weight loss. 2. Reducing diets—Recipes.
3. Self-care, Health.
I. Title. II. Title: Drop ten diet cookbook.
RM222.2.D2732 2013
613.2'5—dc23   2012043557

Photographs by Kana Okada
Food styling by Maggie Ruggiero
Prop Styling by Pam Morris

Printed in the United States of America

www.ballantinebooks.com

246897531

Book design by Casey Hampton

CONTENTS

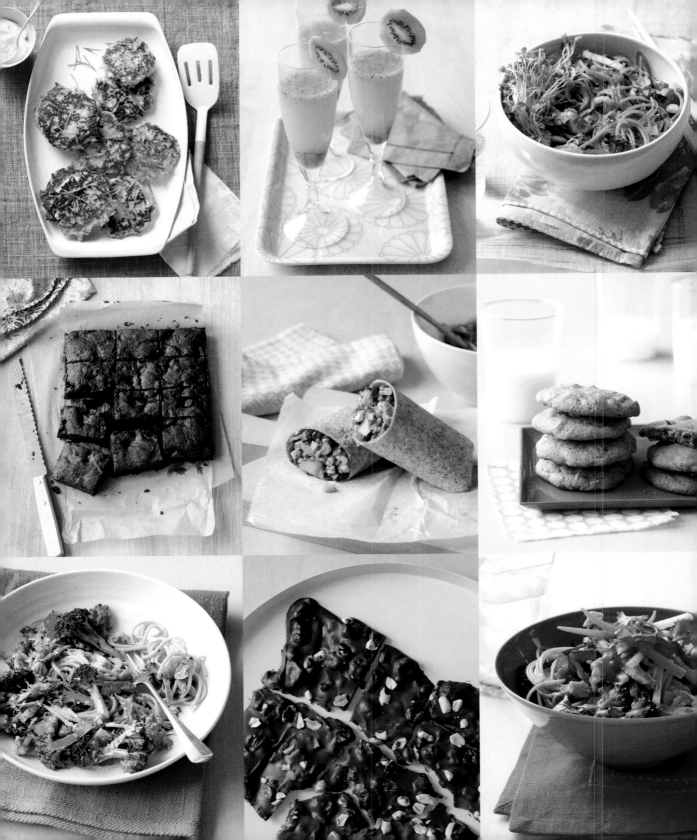

THE
PROGRAM

1 DROP 10, 20, 30+ POUNDS ONE DELICIOUS RECIPE AT A TIME

WHAT IF YOU LEARNED THAT YOU COULD LITERALLY CHANGE your body and your life, one bite at a time? That may sound dramatic, but it's true. The cornerstone of this recipe book is a list of 30 simple, whole foods that science shows can have a significant impact on your weight and health. Each member of this delicious dream team contains nutrients that crank up your metabolism, fill your belly for few calories, stop the cycle of cravings, stymie fat production and storage, and more. Think of these foods as fat-fighting superheroes hiding in plain sight—in the produce aisle, in the dairy case, at the butcher—waiting for you to unleash their pound-peeling power by, well, cleaning your plate.

You may have met these weight loss superfoods in *The Drop 10 Diet,* which featured an easy, repeatable five-week plan to whittle off 10, 20, 30 (or more!) pounds. But even if you didn't, simply swapping some of these recipes into your regular meal rotation can help trigger weight loss. (You can slip them into the easy menu plan in the first book, too.) That's all it takes: Eat more delicious superfoods, lose weight. Study after study, plus our own testers and countless (trimmer!) fans of *The Drop 10 Diet,* have shown that loading up on these nutrition A-listers can improve the odds of weight loss success, help you eat less junk, and pass up the giant portions that pack on flab in the first place.

30 SUPERFOODS FOR WEIGHT LOSS

Almond butter	Eggs	Pomegranates
Apples	Goji berries	Popcorn
Artichokes	Kale	Pumpkin seeds
Avocado	Kiwifruit	Quinoa
Blueberries	Lentils	Sardines
Broccoli	Mushrooms	Steak
Cherries	Oats	Sweet potatoes
Coffee	Olive oil	Whole-grain pasta
Dark chocolate	Parmesan	Wild salmon
Edamame	Peanuts	Yogurt

Before you started reading, you probably already checked out some of the recipes and the luscious-looking photos. At first glance, they may seem to have a lot in common with what many traditional cookbooks offer: tasty crowd-pleasers starring favorites like pasta, steak, cheese, and chocolate. But that's where the similarities end. Not only are these flavorful dishes a snap to make, but each allows you to indulge in the kind of food you love and still lose pounds and inches, lower your risk for major diseases, and gain energy.

THE SUPERFOOD ADVANTAGE

The tasty Drop 10 superfoods offer enough variety to keep you from feeling like a diet zombie, mindlessly feeding on the same lifeless rabbit fare day in and day out. But variety wasn't the only factor we considered when creating the deliciously diverse list. Like instruments in a band or the clothes in your closet, each food brings something cool and different to the table. Here's a sample of what to expect once you begin enjoying the superfood-filled recipes in this book:

- **CALORIES AND BODY FAT WILL DISAPPEAR.** Think about washing a crusty pot with soap and a scrub sponge versus only water and your hand. You'll go through the same motions, but the detergents and sponge make your efforts easier and more effective, and the job goes faster. That's essentially what happens when you eat these superfoods; their nutrients spur you to torch more fat or absorb fewer calories from your meals, so they do a chunk of your weight loss work for you! A few highlights of their stealth power agents:

Calcium blocks fat storage. Eat Parmesan and yogurt and you'll slap down two hormones that otherwise tell your body to pack on fat.

Protein prompts calorie burning. About 100 extra a day, research suggests, if 30 percent of your calories come from this nutrient. Your body has to work harder to digest protein than it does carbs or fat, sizzling up about twice the number of calories in the process. Protein also helps build and maintain lean muscle, which helps rev metabolism (even on those slouch-on-the-couch kind of days).

Healthy fats help strip fat off you. The unsaturated fats in avocado, fish, and olive oil are more readily burned by your body than saturated fats in butter and the like. Researchers aren't sure why, but some suspect that our DNA may be programmed to allow only monounsaturated fat to activate genes that favor fat burning and resist fat storage.

Fiber blocks some calories in food. This body buddy is found in 70 percent of the superfoods (whole-grain pasta, apples, broccoli, even dark chocolate!). If you boost your daily intake to at least 24 grams, you could erase 90 calories a day, a study in *The Journal of Nutrition* reveals. Fiber's trick for making inches disappear: This miracle nutrient binds to some of the fat and calories you eat and directs them through your digestive tract before you absorb them all.

Resistant starch (RS) helps you burn 23 percent more fat. Carbs have a bad rep, but RS is one type you'll want to befriend. It doesn't digest like most other nutrients—instead, it lingers in your system, where it may step up production of hormone compounds that take your flab burning from hot to flaming.

- **YOU'LL THWART YOUR BODY'S PRODUCTION AND STORAGE OF FAT.** The Drop 10 superfoods are digestive slowpokes—and that's a good thing, because as fiber, protein, and fats in food break down, they "feed" your body a slow, steady stream of fuel. Refined carbohydrates (white bread and cookies, for example), full-calorie sodas, and other processed foods digest at a breakneck pace and send a gusher of glucose (your body's main fuel source) into your bloodstream at once. It's more than you need, and the excess gets packed away as fat.

- **HUNGER AND OVEREATING WILL BE DISTANT MEMORIES—ALONG WITH YOUR OLD WAY OF THINKING ABOUT FOOD.** Because they take their time digesting, fiber, protein, and good fats constitute a hunger-quashing, cravings-busting trifecta of trimming. Of the three, protein takes the hunger-taming gold. It decelerates digestion and may enhance the effect of leptin, a key hormone that helps you register fullness. Healthy fats stimulate the release of satiety hormones and are the slowest of the three nutrients to leave your stomach. Omega-3s and resistant starch both may impact hunger and fullness signals, too, and may naturally rein in your appetite. As for fiber, it adds satisfying heft and chewiness to every bite.

- **YOU'LL EAT MORE, YET TAKE IN FEWER CALORIES.** There is another incredibly simple thing that helps hold down hunger: water, found in nearly all of the super fruits and veggies. (Some are up to 92 percent H_2O!) Naturally high water and fiber contents make fruit and veggies low in energy density, meaning you can eat a sizable portion for a decidedly unsizable calorie hit. You'll still feel full; multiple studies show that it's the amount of these foods you eat that satisfies, more so than the actual number of calories you consume.

- **SUPERFOODS NATURALLY CROWD OUT CRUMMY FOODS THAT MAKE YOU FAT.** Unlike most processed foods, the Drop 10 superfoods satisfy you physically and mentally. By swapping out some of your current foods, meals, and drinks for superfood options or simply adding superfoods to what you're already eating, you'll naturally have less room and less desire for the nutritional zeros that add numbers on your scale. No diet drama, no cravings, no calorie math. The only thing you'll count: the pounds as they melt off. It's the ultimate no-diet diet!

SECRETS OF A NO-DIET DIET COOKBOOK

Just as the Drop 10 superfoods aren't traditional "diet" foods, the recipes in this book and in the diet plan you'll read about later in this chapter contain none of the difficult-to-follow hallmarks of trendy programs (banned food groups, weird juices, pricey supplements) or older, overly simplified ones (tasteless servings, calorie counts that couldn't satisfy a toddler). So many diets focus on all the things you *can't* eat—we say, what a drag! Plus, many are so strict, expensive, or time consuming that they're virtually impossible to stick to, making you feel as if *you* failed, when it's the diet that failed you. (So it's no surprise that up to 80 percent of dieters who lose weight can't keep it off!) The easy Drop 10 plan and recipes turn dieting on its head, giving you permission to eat more of what your body craves and setting you up for lifetime success.

Since *The Drop 10 Diet* launched in March 2012, we've heard over and over how the superfoods approach has helped countless people just like you shed 10, 20, even more than 30 pounds, precisely because it eliminates deprivation and instead spotlights the fresh, bursting-with-flavor meals and treats you *can* eat. (You read that right—treats! We'll get to those soon.) A few examples to whet your appetite: Chocolate Chunk and Cherry Pancakes (page 65), Chicken-Fried Flank Steak over Creamy Artichokes with Yogurt and Parmesan (page 131), even Truffled Mac and Cheese (page 98). Yeah, doesn't sound like diet food to us, either! The beauty of this plan also rests in its flexibility with respect to your budget, schedule, social life, and food preferences. By embracing Drop 10 and these recipes, you will give up a few things, however: hunger pangs, cravings, food-induced mood swings, and bland, befuddling recipes. Oh, and the extra weight you're carrying, of course.

Bottom line: This book isn't about being on a diet. Instead, it gives you easy ways to make every forkful work *for* you, with multitasking meals that fuel you up even as they help you slim down to a better body. All you have to do to lose the weight is eat! Here's how the recipes do it:

YOU GET HEARTY PORTIONS, NOT HIDDEN CALORIES. You probably already know that eating out can be a minefield of monster servings and gobs of butter, sugar, and salt. No wonder research shows that the more you dine out, the more likely you are to fill out over time. But undercover calories lurk at home, too. Frozen meals can average 8 percent more calories than what's listed on the box, according to a study in the *Journal of the American Dietetic Association.* Worse, some classic cookbook recipes have become more calorific—soaring an average of 63 percent (between 1936 and 2006), thanks to extra fat, sugar, and bigger portion sizes, find Cornell University researchers.

With supersize servings everywhere you look, you can't be blamed for thinking a sensible portion looks skimpy. The recipes in this book take care of that by featuring plenty of low-energy-dense superfoods that allow you to dig into helpings that are substantial in size only, not calorie load.

YOUR FAVORITE MEALS GET DELICIOUS MAKEOVERS. The average family eats the same nine meals week in and week out, according to a survey by British food company Merchant Gourmet. Some of the favorites—spaghetti Bolognese, pizza, sausage—are also the most likely to cause you to gain weight. In this cookbook, you'll find recipes for these dishes that won't haunt you on the scale later—instead, they'll send the needle in the other direction. Plus, you'll find dozens of tasty options to help you break free of meal monotony, break up the cycle of weight creep, and break out brag-size clothing.

NOT AN EXPERIENCED COOK? YOU CAN STILL MAKE THESE EASY RECIPES. For each dish, the instructions are clear and simple, and they require no *Top Chef*–ready kitchen skills. Nor will we ask you to run around town hunting for hard-to-find ingredients.

Instead, you'll have time to do other things—like shop for skinny jeans. This book delivers fast food like you've never seen it: 16 recipes you can pull together in less than 10 minutes, plus special tags throughout to help you pick out dishes that best meet your needs—those that are kid-friendly, ideal for vegetarians, even no-cook. Meanwhile, chapter 4 is rich with how-to advice for menu planning and ways to make prepping, cooking—and losing—a total cinch.

The only mistake you might make when using this cookbook is thinking "easy" means "boring." Take another flip through the recipes—the inventive dishes and fantastic flavors are both delicious and filling. You know what *is* boring? Stopping at the drive-through again. People who ate at quick-serve spots more than twice a week gained an average of 10 more pounds over 15 years than those who stopped in less than once a week, reports a study in *The Lancet*. Why not use these recipes to curb a fast-food or take-out habit and save yourself some serious poundage?

CHOOSE HOW YOU LOSE

Each recipe provides an optimal balance of hunger-taming, calorie-burning, fat-obliterating nutrients. But how you incorporate them into your routine is your call. (We told you the plan was flexible!) Ready to choose your culinary weight loss adventure?

DROP 10 OPTION 1:
WHIP UP THE DISHES THAT SOUND
MOST DELICIOUS AND WATCH WEIGHT FALL OFF

Do you hate dieting so much you'd rather count cellulite dimples than calories? Want to test-drive the superfoods before committing? Or are you looking for a way to health-ify your current homemade meals for your family? Use this cookbook as you would any other: Pick the recipes that pique your interest and slip them into your usual menu. Or better yet, swap them in for some of the overused, overly caloric dishes currently in your rotation. For example, send that tired tuna casserole back to 1983 and enjoy Quinoa-Crusted Wild Salmon with Broccoli Couscous (page 139) instead. Or save a phone call and dial up your dinner's flavor with homemade Veggie Pad Thai (page 95). By eating more recipes packed with pound-peeling superfoods, you'll automatically trim fat from your body without feeling as if you're overhauling your whole life—or even dieting at all. That's the point. But you will still achieve incredible results—better-fitting clothes, a whittled-down waist, more energy, and an overall feeling of health and well-being. Doesn't that sound good?

DROP 10 OPTION 2:
FOLLOW THE DROP 10 DIET TO LOSE 2 POUNDS PER WEEK

When you've finally had enough of demoralizing deprivation diets, or you're sick and tired (literally!) of being overweight and are ready to take charge of your health, the full Drop 10 plan is a painless way to achieve your better-body goals once and for all. The diet is as straightforward and easy to follow as the recipes in this book: Fill your plate with the superfood-packed breakfasts, lunches, snacks, and dinners on the following pages, sprinkle in your favorite, must-have foods, and let simmer. Add a little exercise and after five weeks, ta-da! You've dropped 10 pounds! Pretty palatable, right? So are the simple details:

Step 1: Eat three squares and a snack daily. Think of each recipe as a block you use to build your base diet of 1,400 calories per day. Don't worry, we've already done the annoying calorie counting for you: The breakfasts are all about 350 calories per serving, lunches and dinners run 450 calories each, and snacks weigh in at 150 calories. Fill up on the recipes that sound best to you, but try to take in a range of the superfoods. Because each one has unique fat-fighting properties, the more you hit, the higher your pounds-off potential.

Step 2: Treat yourself to "happy calories"! On top of your meals and snacks, indulge in up to 200 additional calories daily—yes, we mean candy, ice cream, cocktails, whatever you choose! That's why we call them happy calories—because that's how they make you feel. Allow us to offer a suggestion, though: The superfood-loaded (and delicious) drinks starting on page 191 and desserts on page 201 deliver extra pound-sizzling power that will turn happy calories into bonus whittlers, so you'll enjoy full-on grin-a-thons once you hop on the scale.

But we know 200 calories don't go far when you're, say, celebrating a birthday or out partying with pals. Our solution: Have what you want, of course! You can save up to four days' worth of happy calories (800 in total) and blow them all at once. That calls for a celebration!

Step 3: Go ahead and live your life. We also know that as much as you might like to cook, nobody wants to fix every. single. meal. at. home. So, when you're eating out, look for menu items featuring the superfoods, check the calories on the restaurant's website (or look them up at NutritionData.Self.com), and aim to stay within your day's 1,600 base and happy calorie budget. Easy! You can also follow the menu plan in *The Drop 10 Diet* book, which includes hundreds of fast-food and chain restaurant meal options; find it at major in-store and online retailers.

Whichever route you take, with high-quality fuel in your tank and the freedom to eat the foods you love, you'll start shrinking, yet feel more energized than ever. Maybe even happier and calmer. (Studies show nutrients in some of the superfoods may brighten your mood.) Those positive results beget more healthy behavior, and soon, choosing the right bites and whipping up good-for-you meals will seem natural—as will admiring a slimmer you in the mirror every day. The best part? It can all start now with a single, scrumptious meal.

SPEED UP YOUR WEIGHT LOSS

You can eat your way down to your goal weight if you like, but you'll get there faster if you make regular exercise a habit. (You'll lose about 1 pound a week if you eat a superfood dish at every meal, but double that loss if you work out.) Don't worry—we'd never ask you to put in hours at the gym or master difficult routines. Believe it or not, you can exercise less and trim down faster. The magic trick? Tabata intervals, based on research by a Japanese workout whiz named Izumi Tabata, PhD. Here's the deal: Forget about pushing out the typical two sets of 10 reps per workout. Instead, do a move for 20 seconds, rest for 10, and repeat eight times before you move on to the next exercise. You're done with eight exercises in thirty-two minutes; repeat three times a week. You'll also want to burn off 700 calories a week with cardio—try Zumba, jogging, kickboxing, walking, whatever you like!

Need ideas for moves and cardio workouts? Check *The Drop 10 Diet* for an easy-to-follow plan, or log on to Self.com to find tons of fun routines.

2 MEET THE SUPERFOODS: YOUR POUNDS-OFF PARTNERS FOR LIFE

YOU KNOW THAT MOMENT WHEN YOU LEARN SOMETHING COOL about an acquaintance and it instantly makes you want to be BFFs? Or when a date surprises you with a killer sense of humor and you start planning the wedding in your head? Well, you're about to experience a similar phenomenon thirty times over. After you learn about the superfoods' amazing abilities—to melt fat, incinerate calories, head off cravings, fight disease, and more—you'll never think of them as ordinary foods again. Take that apple sitting in your crisper drawer, for example. Rather than seeing it as a simple snack, you'll recognize it as a fiber-filled force for good. The can of sardines languishing on a pantry shelf? Its belly-flattening powers may make it your go-to salad topper. (No fooling!) And the stash of dark chocolate, prone to inciting guilt and regret? It will lose the devilish horns and grow wings and a halo instead.

That's the point of this chapter. It's not only to excite you with all the science-proven ways the delicious superfoods in these recipes can help you reach your better-body goals. Our primary aim is to compel you to rethink your notions of dieting altogether, to help you understand that food isn't an enemy agent, but an operative that can clear your path to diet and health success. It's only a matter of picking the right ones, and we've done that work for you here. All you have to do is eat them!

HEALTH PERKS OF SUPERFOODS

Along with their slimming powers, eating the superfoods will improve your health, too. Look for these bonus benefits:

BEAUTY BOUNTY: The skin-friendly vitamins, antioxidants, and omega-3 fatty acids in these superfoods promote a gorgeous glow from within.

BONE BUILDER: Calcium-rich foods help build and maintain strong bones.

BRAIN FOOD: Antioxidants, omega-3 fatty acids, and other nutrients in these superfoods help guard against Alzheimer's, elevate your mood, alleviate headaches, and more.

CANCER FIGHTER: Research suggests that certain high-fiber, whole-grain, and antioxidant-rich foods can lower your risk for a variety of cancers.

DIABETES DODGER: Certain superfoods enhance healthy metabolic functioning, possibly lowering your odds of developing this obesity-related disease.

HEART HELPER: These eats help regulate or improve cholesterol, blood pressure, or other cardiovascular risk factors.

IMMUNITY BOOSTER: Rich in probiotics (healthy bacteria that live in your gut), prebiotics (which nourish the good bugs), antioxidants, or other vitamins and minerals, these bites may help you fight off infection.

SIGHT SAVER: These superfoods protect your peepers with potent antioxidants and other nutrients.

TUMMY TAMER: While they are busting belly fat, some superfoods may also help normalize digestion, ease discomfort from GI upsets, or even lessen the severity of menstrual cramps.

Ready to meet your thirty new life partners? They're here to help you become your healthiest, slimmest, best self.

1. ALMOND BUTTER

Slimming secret weapons: fiber, protein, unsaturated fat
Healthy perks: beauty bounty, brain food, heart helper, immunity booster

This rich spread is the cream of the get-trim crop, thanks to a trio of nutrients that work together to edge out hunger and blunt the insulin spikes notorious for turning calories into fat. Fiber-rich foods like almond butter also zip through your digestive system before every calorie can be absorbed, and your body has to burn more calories breaking down protein than it does simple carbs. A milder-tasting version of its peanut counterpart, almond butter also touts higher levels of fat-zapping calcium and energizing iron. Trust us, it's like *buttah*.

CHEF TIPS

- Look for almond butter with only one ingredient—almonds. You won't miss the bloat-causing salt, calorie-adding sugar (aka evaporated cane juice), or saturated-fat-filled palm oil.
- Mix almond butter often to prevent the solids from settling in a tight pack. If that happens, use a steak knife for easy reblending.
- If you prefer whole almonds to the butter, snack away! They contain the same winning combo of weight loss nutrients.

2. APPLES

Slimming secret weapons: fiber, water
Healthy perks: brain food, cancer fighter, heart helper

Weighing in at a juicy 86 percent H_2O, this fruit fills you up, but not with calories. When people munched an apple fifteen minutes before eating a pasta lunch, they took in 187 fewer calories total than those who didn't get the fruit appetizer, a study from Pennsylvania State University at University Park reports. Aside from topping off your tank to prevent overeating, apple's fiber also targets fat: It whisks a portion of what you eat out of your body before you absorb it and stabilizes blood sugar to head off excess fat production.

- All apples are filling and fiber-rich, so go with the variety you like best.
- Keep 'em cool. Apples last longer (three weeks!) in the fridge.
- Savor the skin. Most of apple's fiber and antioxidants live in the peel.

3. ARTICHOKES

Slimming secret weapons: fiber, resistant starch
Healthy perks: cancer fighter, heart helper

When it comes to belly-filling fiber, you can't do much better than these prickly globes. One-half cup of hearts carries 7 grams—more than any other vegetable. Fiber digests slowly to keep you full, plus it ushers some of what you eat out of your body before it can decamp for your thighs. In fact, research shows adding fiber to your diet causes both pounds and body fat to disappear. Artichokes' resistant starch, meanwhile, may trigger the body to burn extra fat and shrink fat cells.

CHEF TIPS

- Fresh chokes make a great snack (see page 47 for prep instructions), but for recipes, use frozen hearts to save time and effort. (Canned and jarred versions tend to be higher in sodium.)
- Choose the right choke. Our superfood, the green globe artichoke, is in a different family altogether from the Jerusalem artichoke (also called a sunchoke).
- Think small. If you come across tiny artichokes, snag a bag. Their size indicates only that they grew lower on the stem, not that they're inferior. With fewer outer leaves and no "hair" hiding the hearts, these babies make for quick prep.

4. AVOCADO

Slimming secret weapons: fiber, monounsaturated fat
Healthy perks: diabetes dodger, heart helper

It's no secret that avocados are full of fat. But that's one reason they're good at helping you *lose* flab. Confused? Don't be: Avocados contain healthy monounsaturated fat, which is filling, spark the production of appetite-regulating hormones, and curtail fat storage. Avocados also have a lot of fiber; half a fruit delivers almost 7 grams.

- The skin of Hass avocados (the most common variety) turns dark when ripe, although other types may not change color. Squeeze before you buy; if there is too much give, move on.
- To keep a cut avocado or guacamole from going brown in the fridge, sprinkle it with lemon juice before storing in an airtight container.

5. BLUEBERRIES

Slimming secret weapons: anthocyanins, fiber
Healthy perks: beauty bounty, brain food, cancer fighter, heart helper, tummy tamer

So sweet to eat, so sweet on the scale: A cup of blueberries packs a filling, trimming 4 grams of fiber into a tiny 84 calories. Berries' anthocyanins—potent antioxidants that give the fruit its rich color—may also set off a skinny-making chain reaction that starts with DNA. Preliminary research suggests they switch on genes that activate proteins known to ramp up fat burning and hinder fat storage.

CHEF TIPS

- The bluer the hue, the riper the fruit. Also look for firm, plump, smooth-skinned orbs; a stained container may indicate overly ripe or moldy berries.
- Rinse the berries right before you eat them; residual moisture may cause them to spoil more quickly.
- Frozen berries are ideal for recipes—keep a bag on hand and you'll always have them when you need them.

6. BROCCOLI

Slimming secret weapons: fiber, vitamin C, water
Healthy perks: beauty bounty, cancer fighter, heart helper, sight saver

Broccoli may seem boring, but then at first glance, so did Clark Kent. Underneath a nerdy exterior, there's superhero power! Weighing in at only 31 calories per chopped cup, the veggie beefs up the volume of meals while helping you shrink. People who ate about three extra servings of low-energy-dense produce daily lost an average of 13 pounds—even though they were taking in about an extra ½ pound of food a day—a study from Pennsylvania State University in University Park reveals. And with more vitamin C than an orange, broccoli encourages your body to make plenty of carnitine, which escorts fat to cells for incineration.

CHEF TIPS

- Seek out dark green florets that are packed close, and bend the stalk gently to test that it's rigid, not rubbery.
- Save the stems: Julienne broccoli stalks and toss them into salads or stir-fries—they're as packed with fiber and nutrients as the florets.
- Broccoli is a perfect freezer staple; microwave a cup or two and toss with pasta, add to soups and stews, or eat as a side dish to feast and still lose flab.

7. CHERRIES

Slimming secret weapons: anthocyanins, fiber
Healthy perks: brain food, cancer fighter, heart helper

Cherries' scarlet hue is more than appealing: Color-adding anthocyanins may trigger enzymes that lead to enhanced fat burning. Animal research from the University of Michigan in Ann Arbor also suggests they improve how the body metabolizes sugar, which helps fight belly fat. In addition, cherries tout fiber and an irresistibly sweet flavor that leave your stomach and your psyche satisfied for a scant 87 calories per cup.

CHEF TIPS

- When buying fresh cherries, skip the gold ones and scoop up the darkest red orbs you can find; they contain the most anthocyanins.
- Tart cherries help you trim down, too, but you typically only find them dried. Choose a bag with no added sweeteners.
- Rinse fresh cherries just before you eat them. As with blueberries, moisture may cause them to spoil swiftly.

8. COFFEE

Slimming secret weapon: caffeine
Healthy perks: brain food, cancer fighter, diabetes dodger, heart helper

Sit, sip, and get slim: The caffeine in coffee boosts your resting metabolic rate—the base number of calories you burn when you're inactive—for up to four hours. Java's buzz might also trigger cells to release fat to torch for energy, and it may prevent muscle fatigue during exercise. Down a cup prior to a sweat session and you may go longer and harder (and blow through more calories), yet not feel any more wiped out. You'll notice the difference, though, when you find your jeans are more roomy than restrictive.

CHEF TIPS

- For the best flavor, grind your beans right before brewing or using in recipes. Coffee gets its flavor from the beans' oils, which degrade quickly.
- To extend the shelf life of beans, stash them in an opaque, airtight container away from heat and light.
- The taste of beans varies regionally, so experiment to find your favorite. African, Caribbean, Hawaiian, and Mexican coffees tend to be lighter; for a fuller-bodied buzz, look to South and other Central American varieties.

9. DARK CHOCOLATE

Slimming secret weapons: cacao, fiber
Healthy perks: beauty bounty, brain food, cancer fighter, heart helper

If there's anything we've learned at *SELF* in our thirty-plus years of reporting on diets and nutrition, it's that deprivation usually backfires. Knowing you're "allowed" to indulge a little helps you resist cravings and avoid binges. But dark chocolate isn't just any old indulgence. It's deeply satisfying, thanks to its naturally intense flavor, plus it boasts 3 grams of filling fiber per 1-ounce serving (for brands with 70 to 80 percent cacao) as well as satiating fat. Also an antioxidant powerhouse, dark chocolate may improve insulin sensitivity and lower levels of the stress hormone cortisol, helping to flatten abs.

- The darker the chocolate, the more slimming. Choose one labeled at least 70 percent cacao.
- Since chocolate is high in calories, limit yourself to an ounce per day when you're eating it plain.
- Try dark chocolate pieces or nibs (whole, shelled cacao beans), which are perfect for cooking and baking.

10. EDAMAME

Slimming secret weapons: choline, fiber, potassium, protein
Healthy perks: bone builder, heart helper

Edamame packs a powerful protein punch, which revs your calorie burn and makes the beans super satiating. And unlike tofu or animal sources of protein, they have 8 grams of fiber per cup, plus bloat-busting potassium. Also rich in the B-vitamin choline, the mighty beans may help block fat absorption and break down fat, too.

CHEF TIPS

- It's rare to find fresh edamame, but the frozen kind is easier to cook with, anyway. And unless it's for snacking, choose the shelled beans.
- If a recipe calls for peas, lima beans, or chickpeas, swap in edamame for extra fat-fighting protein.

11. EGGS

Slimming secret weapons: choline, protein, vitamin D
Healthy perks: beauty bounty, sight saver

No wonder eggs are breakfast staples: They fight body fat with a wallop of hunger-controlling protein and other nutrients that suppress your appetite all day and into the next day, a study in the *Journal of the American College of Nutrition* revealed. And at only 72 calories each (or a barely-there 17 per egg white), it doesn't come at a high cost. You also take in choline, a vitamin that may block fat absorption, and vitamin D; low levels of D are thought to instruct your body to cling to fat, rather than use it for fuel.

CHEF TIPS

- On a budget? Conventional eggs are a healthy bargain. Choose brown or white—there's no nutritional difference.
- If you've got a few extra dollars to spend, consider buying eggs enriched with omega-3 fatty acids—but only if you eat the yolks. They contain all the extra omega-3s.

12. GOJI BERRIES

Slimming secret weapons: fiber, protein, vitamin C
Healthy perks: beauty bounty, cancer fighter, sight saver

If you've never heard of these tart, red-orange fruits, which are typically sold dried, you'll want to try them *stat*. Eighteen amino acids crowd into each tiny berry, giving you 4 grams of satiating, calorie-firing protein per 1-ounce serving. That's as much as an egg! But here's the thing: You also get all the slimming fiber of fruit—about 3 grams per serving—plus about 20 percent of your day's quota for vitamin C, which helps your body burn fat.

CHEF TIPS

- Find gojis stocked with other dried fruit in the produce department or snack food section. If your supermarket doesn't carry them, order online.

13. KALE

Slimming secret weapons: fiber, vitamin C
Healthy perks: beauty bounty, brain food, cancer fighter, heart helper

Like its green buddy broccoli, kale is one of the best low-energy-dense foods available. At only 34 calories per cup, kale lets you cut back on calories without leaving you hungry. Fiber makes it filling, and it blocks absorption of some of the fat you eat in other foods. One cup of kale also feeds you more than a day's worth of vitamin C, which helps make fat available to cells that burn it for energy.

- Kale is commonly found in two varieties: Curly kale has ruffled leaves, a rigid stem, and a strong flavor, while Tuscan kale (aka lacinato or dinosaur) has flat, textured leaves and a milder taste.
- The freshest bunch sports dark green leaves that look firm and crisp.
- Store kale in an open plastic bag in the coldest part of your fridge and eat within a few days—it gets bitter over time.

14. KIWIFRUIT

Slimming secret weapons: fiber, potassium, vitamin C
Healthy perks: beauty bounty, cancer fighter, heart helper, immunity booster, tummy tamer

What's so cool about kiwi? That such a small fruit is so big on nutrition and fat-fighting power. One kiwi contains more than a day's worth of vitamin C, which may help maximize fat burning during exercise. People with low levels burned about 10 percent less fat per pound of body weight while walking compared with those in the normal range, research from Arizona State University reveals. Kiwi also fits fiber and potassium into its petite package, all for a bikini-friendly 42 calories.

CHEF TIPS

- Gently press a kiwi before buying. A ripe one feels soft but not mushy. Let hard fruit ripen at room temperature before refrigerating.
- Leave prep to the last minute: Kiwi's flesh contains an enzyme that acts as a food tenderizer when exposed to air, turning the fruit and other food it touches mushy.
- Love the fuzz. The skin is edible and loaded with fiber.

15. LENTILS

Slimming secret weapons: fiber, protein, resistant starch
Healthy perks: beauty bounty, cancer fighter, diabetes dodger, heart helper, tummy tamer

No beans about it, lentils are top-notch waist whittlers. With more fiber than most other foods—16 grams per cup—they fill you up quickly, then digest at a pokey pace that keeps insulin levels steady and saves calories from a fatty fate. Lentils' protein helps satiate you, too, while its resistant starch may help burn fat. The evidence is convincing: Dieters who ate lentils and other legumes four times a week lost 54 percent more weight than those who followed a low-cal plan without the fat fighters, researchers at the University of Navarra in Pamplona, Spain, report.

CHEF TIPS

- Lentils come in a variety of types and colors; brown lentils are the most common. Inexpensive and versatile, they tend to hold their shape well.
- Red lentils break down easily, making them an ideal addition to creamy soups and stews. They look orange or salmon pink in the bag and turn yellow or gold after cooking.
- Don't feel like cooking lentils? Hit up the refrigerated veggie section to find pre-cooked, ready-to-eat bags.

16. MUSHROOMS

Slimming secret weapons: umami, water
Healthy perks: cancer fighter, heart helper, immunity booster

Eating fewer calories than you burn is weight loss 101. The advanced lesson: Choosing low-energy-dense foods means you can do it sans hunger. With just a handful of calories (thanks to a 92 percent water content), fungi are great at bulking up meals, not your body. But unlike other low-energy-dense foods, mushrooms' soft, thick texture and savory flavor (called umami) make them seem meaty. Swap them for ground beef in recipes and you save calories and fat without sacrificing satisfaction.

CHEF TIPS

- All mushrooms help you slim, so if there's one type you like best, eat that. Buttons (white mushrooms) are most common and among the lowest in calories (15 per chopped cup). Portobello and cremini (baby bella) taste earthier and deliver 22 and 19 calories per chopped cup, respectively.
- Look for packages of mushrooms that brag about extra vitamin D. It means manufacturers set them under sunlamps, which boost levels of the nutrient.

- Don't soak or rinse 'shrooms; wipe away soil and residue with a damp cloth to preserve the flavor.

17. OATS

Slimming secret weapon: fiber
Healthy perks: brain food, diabetes dodger, heart helper, immunity booster

All whole grains fill you up with belly-trimming fiber, but oats deliver a special form called beta-glucan, which digests slowly to control fat-making insulin spikes also seems to switch on hormones that control hunger. That may help explain why oatmeal is one of the most satiating foods you can eat. Oats' fiber may also quell inflammation in your body, possibly helping you sidestep metabolic syndrome, a condition characterized by excess belly fat.

CHEF TIPS

- Steel yourself for slimming: Unlike old-fashioned or instant oats, which are rolled flat, the steel-cut variety (sometimes called Scotch or Irish oats) net a heartier, chewier bowl of oatmeal.
- If you prefer instant oats, bypass flavored varieties, which often contain heaps of added sugar. Sweeten with fiber-rich fruit instead.
- Make your own flour. Oat flour, which several of the recipes in this book call for, is considered a specialty product and, as such, comes with a special price tag. But you can make your own by grinding old-fashioned oats in a (clean) coffee grinder for about thirty seconds. One cup of oats yields ¾ cup flour.

18. OLIVE OIL

Slimming secret weapon: monounsaturated fat
Healthy perks: brain food, cancer fighter, diabetes dodger, heart helper

Eating and cooking with olive oil is like filling your gas tank with premium fuel. Rich in monounsaturated fats that help you resist belly flab, olive oil also helps stifle your appetite. One study published in the *British Journal of Nutrition* found that people whose fat came mostly from monounsaturated sources lost weight and body fat over four weeks without making any other changes to their eating habits; a group that ate more saturated fat *gained* in both categories.

- Use extra-virgin olive oil (EVOO) to drizzle on salads and other cold dishes; made from the best olives, it is the most flavorful variety and highest in antioxidants.
- Reach for less expensive light olive oil (aka pure) for baking and cooking. Its neutral flavor works best for muffins, quick breads, and the like. It also stands up to a hot skillet better than EVOO.
- Make a slimming cooking spray by pouring olive oil into a stainless-steel spray bottle. Two pumps will coat a skillet or salad for only about 40 calories.

19. PARMESAN

Slimming secret weapons: calcium, protein
Healthy perks: beauty bounty, bone builder

Cheese gets a bad diet rap, but—like chocolate—it can be a smart indulgence that may help you cut body fat. One ounce provides a third of your daily calcium needs (336 milligrams); once you hit 1,000 milligrams, you can suppress two hormones that otherwise prompt your body to store fat. The cheese also adds 10 grams of satiating protein to any dish, revving up your post-meal calorie burn.

CHEF TIPS

- To get the most flavorful bang for your calorie buck, upgrade from pre-grated sprinkles to a hunk of fresh Parmesan. Ask the cheese monger to grate it or shred it yourself.
- When adding Parm to recipes, use shredded—it melts more easily, and a 1-ounce portion (about ¼ cup) will go farther.

20. PEANUTS

Slimming secret weapons: fiber, monounsaturated fat, protein
Healthy perks: beauty bounty, brain food, diabetes dodger, heart helper

When you're shopping, an 11 percent discount sounds good, right? That's sort of what you'll get by eating these nuts; the snack may boost your metabolism by up to 11 percent, cutting their calorie cost. Experts aren't sure why, although they do know that each nut is a calorie-sizzling protein powerhouse, that your body more readily torches peanuts' healthy monounsaturated fat than it does saturated fat, and that the fiber in the nuts prevents you from absorbing some calories. All this, plus peanuts are aces at silencing hunger.

CHEF TIPS

- Choose raw or dry-roasted, unsalted peanuts to avoid a load of bloating sodium. Also check ingredients lists on labels to be sure sugar isn't tagging along.
- Individual nuts not your thing? Spread the butter instead. But opt for a natural variety that contains only peanuts.
- If a recipe calls for chopped peanuts, don't use your coffee grinder or you may damage the motor. Use a food processor or chopper, or place a handful in a freezer bag and go to town with a meat tenderizer.

21. POMEGRANATE

Slimming secret weapon: fiber
Healthy perks: brain food, cancer fighter, heart helper

If all you know about pomegranates is juice, you're in for a treat. Underneath the fruit's red skin you'll find hundreds of tiny, crunchy, juice-filled seeds (called arils) bursting with sweetness and fat-slashing fiber. While the bright bites are as satisfying and fun to pop as jelly beans, they are the antithesis to sugary candy in your body: Pomegranates' fiber slows digestion, keeping insulin levels steady—and you steadily losing weight. And thanks to a high water content, a filling ½ cup of arils nets you only 72 calories.

CHEF TIPS

- Sold already ripe, whole pomegranates will stay fresh for up to three months if you stash them in a plastic bag in the fridge.
- To save prep time, look for containers of preshucked arils in your grocer's produce section.
- If a recipe calls for pomegranate juice, use one that contains no added sugar and only pom juice. Some brands are juice blends—check the small print on back.

22. POPCORN

Slimming secret weapon: fiber
Healthy perks: beauty bounty, cancer fighter, diabetes dodger, heart helper

Surprise! Popcorn is a weight-whittling whole grain disguised as a fun snack food. Unlike refined grains, which are stripped of their good-for-you nutrients, wholes contain lots of satiating fiber; dieters who ate five servings of whole grains lost more belly flab than those who cut calories but ate refined carbs, according to a study in *The American Journal of Clinical Nutrition*. Hold the oil and butter, and dig into 3 cups of the air-popped variety: You'll take in only 93 calories and no saturated fat.

CHEF TIPS

- Pop for less! Buying a bag of kernels rather than the microwave variety saves you money and calories, since you control the type and amount of flavorings you add. If you don't have an air popper, don't worry; we'll tell you how to prep the corn on page 49.
- If you buy microwavable popcorn, compare labels to find the brands lowest in fat and sodium.

23. PUMPKIN SEEDS

Slimming secret weapons: fiber, protein, unsaturated fat
Healthy perks: brain food, diabetes dodger, heart helper

The best way to quiet hunger, avoid cravings, and melt flab: Make sure your bites contain a combo of protein, fiber, and healthy fats. Pumpkin seeds do this automatically: One ounce delivers 8 grams of protein, which supercharges your calorie burning; 2 grams of fiber to help lower your day's overall calorie haul; and enough healthy fats to keep you full and satisfied.

CHEF TIPS

- Pick pepitas. Opt for pre-hulled (and unsalted) seeds, sometimes called pepitas.
- Store your seeds in an airtight container in the refrigerator and they'll stay fresh for up to six months.

24. QUINOA

Slimming secret weapons: fiber, protein, resistant starch
Healthy perks: beauty bounty, cancer fighter, diabetes dodger, heart helper, tummy tamer

This truly great grain (actually a seed), pronounced *KEEN-wah,* has a light, fluffy texture and nutrients that will help you lighten up, too. Flush with filling fiber and richer in protein than most other whole grains, it delivers a long-term stream of energy, not the insulin spike-and-slump that leaves you dragging and packs on fat. And since it takes longer to digest, protein keeps your body burning calories after you eat.

CHEF TIPS

- Not familiar with the grain? Supermarkets typically stock it in the same aisle as pasta and rice, or in the health or natural food section.
- Rinse first. Quinoa, which you prepare in the same way as rice, has a natural, bitter-tasting coating; a quick rinse prior to cooking lets the mild, nutty flavor shine.

25. SARDINES

Slimming secret weapons: calcium, omega-3 fatty acids, protein, vitamin D
Healthy perks: beauty bounty, bone builder, brain food, heart helper, sight saver

These swimmers are a diet catch: Highly concentrated in omega-3s, which fight belly flab and may rouse enzymes that promote fat burning, sardines also pack satiating, calorie-torching protein (23 grams per 3.75-ounce serving). What's more, they're a good non-dairy source of calcium, thanks to their soft, edible bones.

CHEF TIPS

- Try them! Far from the slimy, stinky image that may be in your head, canned sardines in water taste mild—and similar to tuna. Rinse before using to cut the sodium.
- Fresh sardines taste and smell only slightly briny, even less so than canned. (If you catch one with a strong odor, throw it back.)

- You buy fresh sardines whole, but your fishmonger can clean them for you if you ask.

26. STEAK

Slimming secret weapons: iron, protein
Healthy perks: beauty bounty, immunity booster

The meaty details on steak's diet power: It's all about protein. Multiple studies suggest that getting 25 to 35 percent of your calories from the nutrient helps you lose weight and body fat. Protein fills you up, stabilizes insulin levels, and provides building material for the lean muscle that keeps your metabolism humming on high. Steak also contains iron, which keeps *you* humming—the mineral helps red blood cells carry energizing oxygen.

CHEF TIPS

- Round, sirloin, tenderloin (aka filet mignon), and flank steaks are the skinniest cuts. Always opt for a select grade, which has less fat than prime or choice. Buying ground beef? Pick one that's at least 90 percent lean.
- Go with grass-fed. By far the most diet-friendly type of red meat, grass-fed varieties contain lower amounts of saturated fat and more healthy omega-3s.

27. SWEET POTATOES

Slimming secret weapons: fiber, resistant starch
Healthy perks: beauty bounty, cancer fighter, heart helper

Upgrade your spuds to these diet dynamos and you'll downsize in a jiffy. With more fiber and nutrients than their white counterparts, sweet potatoes help stave off the insulin spikes that trigger fat production and cravings, plus help move food through your digestive system, disposing of it before you absorb all its fat and calories. Sweet potatoes also deliver a special type of carbohydrate that, unlike other starches, resists digestion and instead helps regulate your appetite, shrinks fat cells, and may increase fat and calorie burning.

- Select a spud with smooth, clean skin and a plump shape.
- Sweet potatoes and yams deliver the same benefits, but the latter may have a softer texture when cooked.
- If you're short on time, use canned sweet potatoes in recipes, but only those with no salt, sugar, or other additives.

28. WHOLE-GRAIN PASTA

Slimming secret weapons: fiber, protein, resistant starch
Healthy perks: beauty bounty, brain food, cancer fighter, diabetes dodger, heart helper

Unlike white pasta, whole-grain noodles hang on to their grain's bran and germ, doubling (even tripling!) the amount of fiber you take in, while also delivering a nice dose of protein. Both nutrients effortlessly erase some calories from your day's slate—protein burns extra calories during digestion, and fiber ferries them out of the body before absorption. Resistant starch in the pasta may enhance fullness signals between the gut and brain, as well as prompting fat burning and discouraging fat storage.

CHEF TIPS
- Whole wheat isn't your only whole-grain option; you'll find pasta made from barley, brown rice, buckwheat, durum wheat, kamut, quinoa, rye, spelt, or a blend of a few. All have slightly different textures, so experiment to see which you like best.
- If your pasta package doesn't state "100 percent whole grain" or "whole wheat," check labels and ingredients lists to ensure that the word *whole* precedes each grain listed.
- Although they more closely resemble rice, couscous and orzo are pasta and are available in whole-grain versions.

29. WILD SALMON

Slimming secret weapons: omega-3 fatty acids, protein, vitamin D
Healthy perks: beauty bounty, brain food, cancer fighter, heart helper, sight saver

Think of wild salmon's omega-3s as alpha fats—they take the top diet spot. Research suggests they impact signals that direct your body to sizzle rather than store fat, especially during exercise, plus they help regulate metabolism, curb the munchies, and improve how your body uses sugar. Salmon's omega-3s have a couple of useful sidekicks: vitamin D, which may tame fat-producing hormones, and supersatiating, calorie-blazing protein.

CHEF TIPS

- Although it's slightly more expensive, wild Alaskan or Pacific salmon is lower in contaminants and safer for the environment than the farmed Atlantic variety.
- No matter what form your salmon takes—smoked (called lox), canned, or fresh—you'll still net plenty of pound-shucking nutrients.
- When you freeze fresh salmon, wrap fillets in plastic wrap first, then store in a plastic bag or airtight container to prevent freezer burn.

30. YOGURT

Slimming secret weapons: calcium, protein
Healthy perks: bone builder, tummy tamer

Digging into this low-fat hero alerts belly fat that its days are numbered. One 8-ounce serving contains almost half of your day's calcium needs. Upping your intake of the mineral to at least 1,000 milligrams per day helps your body fend off fat, especially around your middle. That hotshot move, along with yogurt's payload of protein—which doffs hunger, helps stabilize blood sugar, and revs metabolism—makes the creamy treat a powerful tool in your diet arsenal.

CHEF TIPS

- Greek yogurt contains about twice as much protein as regular, and because it's thicker, it works especially well as a slimming substitute for sour cream or mayo. But you'll sacrifice some calcium, so aim to eat both types.
- Compared with nonfat yogurt, low-fat contains only about 10 to 20 more calories per serving, but it may taste a little richer. The Drop 10 recipes call for both types, but you can use them interchangeably.
- For smoothies or other recipes that incorporate yogurt, bypass the sugary fruit and vanilla varieties and choose plain.

3 SET YOURSELF UP FOR SUCCESS

YOU COULD BE AS DEDICATED TO WINNING AT WEIGHT LOSS as an Iron Chef is to ruling Kitchen Stadium, but without the right tools and setup, success may elude you. (No Iron Chef would work the arena with just a butter knife and hot plate, after all!) Prepping your kitchen and pantry will make cooking the superfoods easier, faster, and more fun—and all but guarantees a triumphant victory in your battle with body fat.

YOUR KITCHEN MAKEOVER

Where you prep and cook can have a significant impact on your eating (and overeating) habits. The steps here detail exactly how to stock and streamline your kitchen space for optimal slimming. Don't worry, it's easy! All you have to do is follow along.

STEP 1: TAKE OUT THE TRASH

A fashion makeover starts with a ceremonial toss of clothes that no longer fit your life, and that's how to approach the food you typically keep on hand. You cannot build a healthy diet on the foundation of whatever caused you to pack on pounds in the first place. Don't think of this clean-out as saying good-bye to the foods you love—remember, you get to keep your favorite treats in the mix. Rather, this is the first step toward saying good-bye to excess weight for good.

Set aside an afternoon for the job and tackle one area of the kitchen at a time. Literally pick up and hold each item and ask yourself if it is going to help you reach your goal, using the following guidelines to help you decide what to toss as you go.

TRASH (OR DONATE) THESE FOODS:

Packaged items with long ingredients lists. In general, keep foods with lists that read like a children's book—short and containing only words you recognize. Specifically, check labels for sugar and its evil twins, high-fructose corn syrup and evaporated cane juice. (The suffix *-ose* is also typically code for sugar.) Keep added sugars under 10 grams per serving; the exception is dairy, which has naturally occurring sweet stuff. Also toss foods with partially hydrogenated oils (trans fat in disguise).

Most frozen dinners and canned soup. Even low-calorie and low-fat varieties tend to load you up with sodium (hello, belly bloat) while skimping on portions. Make your own skinnier, tastier, and more satiating versions instead! (Check out "5 Tips to Make Your Own Frozen Meals," page 32.) If you still want to keep prefab grabs around, pick frozen dinners with no more than 700 milligrams of sodium and no more than 4 grams of saturated fat, but with at least 5 grams of fiber and 8 grams of protein. Soups should contain no more than 500 milligrams sodium per serving and feature no added sugar.

Saucy frozen veggies. Both your tush and taste buds will thank you if you sprinkle on fresh Parmesan or zesty spices (see page 35) instead of eating the sauce-drenched fat and sodium bombs from the freezer section. Plain frozen veggies are fine if fresh isn't an option—in fact, since they're picked at peak and iced quickly, frozen produce is super nutritious.

Simple carbohydrates. White bread, bagels and rice, refined (white) pasta, cereal, and other processed grains have been stripped of their slimming fiber and protein. Here's what your body thinks when you eat them: *Sugar! Sugarsugarsugar! More sugar!* And then: *Ugh, too much sugar.* At which point it begins steering those calories into fat.

Foods made with MSG. Also check ingredients lists for monosodium glutamate, hydrolyzed soy protein, or autolyzed yeast. Research from the University of North Carolina at Chapel Hill suggests there may be a link between MSG intake and weight gain, possibly because the additive interferes with your body's appetite signals.

- Undercook the veggies to ensure they maintain some crunch after reheating. Sayonara, sogginess!
- Let food cool in the fridge before freezing to prevent bacteria buildup.
- Store food in smaller containers (single or double servings) to keep portion size reasonable.
- Leave an inch of space between the food and lid of a storage container, since soups and sauces expand during the freezing process.
- Write down what the dish is and the date you froze it on masking tape and stick it on the lid.

Bar food. No, not what you're thinking! We're talking about protein, snack, and meal replacement bars—some healthy-sounding ones are just glorified candy.

Packaged pastries, muffins, and other baked goods. Even low-calorie versions are full of preservatives and artificial sweeteners, which may cause insulin levels to rise, switching on your appetite.

"Diet" products. Many reduced-calorie and low-fat crackers, cheese, muffins, and other items contain preservatives and hunger-promoting sugar substitutes, and they tend to be less satisfying than the real thing, so you may end up eating more.

Superfood imposters. Yogurt-covered raisins sound like a version of a Drop 10 superfood, right? Not so. The coating often contains a mix of added sugars, partially hydrogenated oils, and milk or yogurt powders. Bottom line, as with any packaged food: Always check ingredients lists to get the full story.

STEP 2: BUILD YOUR HEALTHY STASH

Now that you've made a lot of extra room on your shelves, fill it with eats that will get you closer to your goal with every bite.

STOCK THESE SLIM-DOWN HELPERS:

Your favorite treats. Surprised? Remember, we told you that you don't have to give up foods you love! But you don't want to overdo, and the secret is to limit your options. Studies consistently show that variety can trigger people to eat more. So decide which one or two goodies make you happiest—pick one kind of cookie versus three, for instance, or one flavor of ice cream rather than five—and put them in opaque containers out of easy reach.

Whole foods. If it comes in the package Mother Nature designed, it's a keeper. Fruits and veggies are the stars. Along with your usual favorites, stock up on lemons and limes; their juice and zest lend dishes acidity and flavor but few to no calories and zero sodium.

Whole-grain pasta and cereal. Label language can be tricky here; even if a product sounds healthy, check the ingredients lists. The word *whole* should appear in front of any grain you see there. (*Whole grain* or *whole wheat* should also appear first on the list of ingredients, or first after water.)

Whole-wheat pastry flour. Most of our baked goods recipes call for this soft flour, which gives muffins and cakes a light, fluffy texture. Make sure the label reads "pastry flour" (Arrowhead Mills is one brand); regular whole-wheat flour can make your muffins dense and hard.

Oat flour. You'll see this versatile superfood ingredient in several Drop 10 recipes. Rather than shelling out for a bag, make it as you need it by grinding a few batches of old-fashioned rolled oats in a clean coffee grinder and storing it in a plastic zipper bag in the fridge for up to three months, or in the freezer for up to a year. (Even though oats and regular flour stay fresh in the cupboard, grinding releases oats' oils, which turn rancid quickly if left out.)

Fat-free, low-sodium chicken broth or stock. Use these as a base for soups and stews; the latter is seasoned, the former is not. Either way, check labels for sodium levels and aim for less than 450 milligrams per cup.

Canned, diced tomatoes. This diet-friendly staple can turn just about anything into a filling, fat-trimming soup, stew, or pasta sauce on the fly. Opt for an unseasoned can that's free of added sugar and low in sodium (less than 270 mg per ½ cup), so *you* decide whether to go Italian by adding oregano and basil, Mexican by mixing in chile-pepper-based spices, Indian by sprinkling in curry, and so on.

Tomato paste. The concentrated version of versatile diced tomatoes, tomato paste delivers bushels of flavor, few calories, and little sodium.

Low-sodium soy sauce. Give a few shakes to add a distinctive savory flavor to dishes and negate the need for the saltshaker.

Dijon mustard. This condiment provides flavor and binds together oil and vinegar in homemade vinaigrette dressings.

Bulb garlic. Skip the jars of pre-minced garlic, which tend to taste strong and stale and can overpower your dish.

Oils. Healthy fats help stabilize insulin levels, fill you up, and add flavor and a satisfying texture to your dishes. The following oils contain among the highest levels of good-for-you (and your waistline) monounsaturated fats:

- *Extra-virgin olive oil.* EVOO is best used on cooked foods or those that don't require cooking, since the delicate, flavorful oil burns easily. Drizzle it over veggies or salads, and use it in sandwiches instead of mayo or butter.
- *Light olive oil.* With a milder, neutral taste and a higher smoke point than EVOO (meaning it stands up to hotter temperatures before burning), light or pure olive oil is ideal for baking and when you're sautéing, stir-frying, or searing.
- *Olive oil cooking spray.* Spritzing skillets and baking dishes prevents food from sticking and fat and calories from accumulating. For stovetop cooking, heat your skillet first and pull it off the stove before you spray to avoid flare-ups. Then immediately return it to the heat and add food—the spray may burn if left on its own too long.
- *Canola oil (expeller-pressed).* Canola has a higher smoke point than even light olive oil, but it's also rich in healthy monounsaturated fats. Keep some handy for when you really fire up the stove, such as for popping popcorn.

Vinegar. You might catch more flies with honey, but you'll lose more flab by adding this tart ingredient to your diet. Vinegar's acetic acid activates a gene that helps break down fat before it ends up stored in your body. Plus, it may help curb your appetite by hindering hunger-inducing spikes in blood sugar, a study from Lund University in Sweden shows. The four types of vinegar you'll use most often in these recipes:

- *Balsamic.* Although it's not a wine vinegar, balsamic is made from grape pressings, giving it a slightly sweet taste that complements both desserts and savory dishes. (Check labels to be sure your balsamic actually comes from grapes—some brands don't.) Try simmering the vinegar until reduced by half for a syrupy sauce that turns fresh fruit, ice cream, or grilled pork into a gourmet dish.
- *Apple cider.* With its versatile, sweet flavor, apple cider is a budget-friendly stand-in for pricey rice vinegar in Asian dressings and dishes.
- *Red and white wine.* Vino-based vinegars make delicious additions to salad dressings and marinades. For a tummy-trimming vinaigrette, whisk together equal parts red wine vinegar and olive oil, then add a bit of Dijon mustard, plus garlic, salt, and pepper.

- *Hot sauce.* Try a few different chile-based sauces to find the ones that light your fire. Louisiana Hot Sauce and Cholula are blended with Cajun or Mexican seasonings, respectively, while Sriracha and sambal heat up Asian flavors. And as for good old Tabasco? It's a spicy chameleon; add a few dashes to pasta dishes, veggies, sandwiches, hummus, mayo—anything! It even turns orange juice into a sweet-and-spicy treat.

Herbs and spices. When overweight people sprinkled dishes with flavor enhancers, they lost significantly more weight over six months than those who didn't, according to a study from the Smell & Taste Treatment and Research Foundation in Chicago. The flavor agents practically insist that you focus on the taste and smell of food, helping you feel satiated sooner. Plus, capsaicin, the compound that makes chiles hot (it's in hot sauces, red pepper flakes, and chili powders), fires up your metabolism.

Herbs' flavor potency comes from delicate oils that can degrade the longer they sit on your shelf. Using fresh stuff when possible ensures the freshest-tasting food. You can grow your own to save money; if space is tight, a sunny windowsill is all you need. (Check out "Save Calories and Cash," page 36, for simple how-tos. For ideas on what to sprinkle on your meals, see "Your Slimming Spice Rack," below.)

YOUR SLIMMING SPICE RACK

Black peppercorns	Dill	Paprika
Cayenne pepper	Fine-grain sea salt	Red pepper flakes
Chili powder	Garlic powder	Rosemary
Cinnamon	Ginger	Sage
Cumin	Madras curry powder	Thyme
Curry powder	Oregano	Turmeric

TIPS FOR SENSATIONAL, SLIMMING SEASONING

- Crack black pepper as you use it; peppercorns contain oils that, when pre-milled, degrade quickly and can devolve into a dusty taste.
- Just ¼ teaspoon of cinnamon may prevent the fat-storing spikes in insulin that can occur after you eat.
- Fine-grain sea salt adds robust flavor to meals, allowing you to sprinkle less salt than you would from a regular shaker.

A small herb garden on your deck, fire escape, or windowsill provides fresh, flab-melting flavor on the cheap. Get growing!

Plot your pots. The following herbs are hardy enough to flourish in small spaces: basil, chives (which you can sub for green onions), dill, mint, oregano, tarragon, rosemary, and thyme. You could grow cilantro and parsley, too, but both are usually inexpensive and readily available at the supermarket.

Skip the seeds. Use starter plants to save you time. Repot into 5- to 8-inch vessels with potting soil to give them room to grow; make sure there is a hole in the bottom to facilitate drainage or the roots may rot. Since basil typically takes up more space than other herbs as it grows (and you'll use more of it), combine a few starter plants in one 10-inch-diameter (or larger) pot. For all, wait to plant until you're sure the weather won't dip below 45°F, or bring them inside at night.

Find some sun. Most herbs require sun to grow, but avoid areas that get direct sun from morning to night without reprieve.

Water in the early evening. If you do it in the morning, wet soil can bake in the sun and harden, which can hurt your herbs. Also avoid drowning your plants—aim for slightly moist soil, not puddles.

Harvest sparingly. When you clip sprigs and leaves for cooking, always leave enough of the plant behind to support regrowth.

- Chunky and oily, ground chili powder mixes well with whole-wheat bread crumbs for a dry rub, since it doesn't burn on a hot pan as other spices can.
- Paprika adds mild, smoky heat to food, and a deep beautiful red shade.
- Use red pepper flakes to spice up pizza, pasta, cooked veggies, and salad. Adding it to food may prompt you to take in fewer calories and less fat at subsequent meals, a study in the *British Journal of Nutrition* reports.

STEP 3: DECLUTTER YOUR KITCHEN

If you have to spend ten minutes restacking the mail and clearing away to-do lists, newspapers, your laptop, kids' art projects, and countless other items just to find your counter and dining table, it's no wonder you end up reaching for take-out menus instead of cooking. Starting today, declare your kitchen a no-clutter zone; anything non-food-related that comes in must quickly be dealt with or stashed elsewhere. Set aside a basket or a drawer where you can put papers and other items you may want in the kitchen but which don't need to be on the kitchen table and counter.

STEP 4: ARRANGE YOUR SPACE FOR SLIMMING

Consider this step the lipstick phase of your kitchen's makeover—the finishing touch that can elevate results from so-so to sensational. The key to organizing: Whatever is most visible will dictate what you eat. Try these streamlining tactics:

In the fridge and freezer. Countless fruits and veggies have died slow deaths in crisper drawers. Move 'em on up to a higher shelf where they will be the first things you lay eyes on when opening the door. The same goes for the freezer: Stash ice cream on the bottom or hidden in the back, and place frozen fruit and veggies at eye level.

In your pantry and cupboards. Nuts and nut butter, dried fruit, whole-grain crackers, canned vegetables, oatmeal, quinoa, sardines—seeing these types of foods first can help stop mindless snacking and overeating before it starts by subtly suggesting you fill up on healthier, more filling fare.

On and around kitchen counter. Keep cutting boards and your chef's knives out and near each other; they can serve as a reminder to eat produce and cook more often. Chopping may also feel like less of a chore if your tools are readily accessible. The same goes for items such as a blender and skillet. Consider getting a magnetic knife holder for the wall above your counter and a hanging rack for pots and pans.

THINK SMALL

Shopping at warehouse clubs can save you money, but may cost you on the scale. People tend to consume ready-to-eat food faster when they buy it in bulk, according to research from Brian Wansink, PhD, professor of marketing at Cornell University. Likewise, we tend to gobble more ready-to-eat foods when reaching into bigger boxes and bags. Transfer whatever you buy in bulk into smaller, refillable containers that you keep out of sight and replenish as needed.

What if you had a gadget that could instantly open up an express lane during rush hour? Or one that turned a tedious task like folding laundry into a fun game? That's essentially what the right kitchen tools do. They facilitate your flab-melting mission by making food prep easy, quick, and fun and by helping your meals taste (and look!) delicious. Stocking your culinary Bat Cave is easy: Below you'll find a list of basic items, along with tips on how to use them, where you can penny-pinch, and why some splurge-worthy items are worth it. Now, chef, ready to meet your kitchen staff?

BEST COOKWARE AND BAKEWARE

Pots and pans are a home cook's bread and butter. Chances are you already own some of these, but you may want to consider an upgrade.

A large and medium skillet or sauté pan. High-quality stainless steel conducts heat well and evenly, helping food cook perfectly. You'll be using skillets often, and the material is oven- and dishwasher-safe and cleans up easily. So if there's any category that's worth the splurge, this is it. All-Clad brand, the cream of the crop and a favorite among chefs, runs $100 for a large, 11-inch size; or you can get a five-piece set (two pans, a sauce pot, and lids) for about $350. Pricey, yes, but chances are you'll be passing them down to your kids. Bargain versions, on the other hand, are notorious for burning food and can be hard to clean. And nonstick skillets can lose their coating after a few years and aren't safe in the dishwasher or oven. Besides, a little cooking spray turns stainless steel virtually nonstick anyway—even when you're frying eggs.

Sauce pot. Stainless steel reigns supreme here, too. But it's okay to skimp on a pot since it sees much less action than a skillet. A 1½- or 2-quart size is handy when making or warming up small batches of sauce, noodles, and soup.

Large soup pot. An inexpensive stainless-steel 4-quart soup or stew pot will do the trick, but if you can spend more, consider a heavy, enamel-coated cast-iron Dutch oven or pot, which you can also use in the oven. Amateur and pro chefs covet the Le Creuset pot, which costs about $240 for a 4½-quart size but lasts a lifetime or longer. It conducts heat perfectly and, thanks in part to its heft and heavy lid, holds and cooks liquids in a way that seamlessly blends flavors.

Muffin tins and cookie sheets. This is one category where we recommend you spend less. Yep, our chef actually prefers the inexpensive, uncoated bakeware you can buy at the grocery store. The metal heats and cooks well and evenly, whereas pricier nonstick varieties may burn muffin and cookie bottoms. And—bonus!—the bakeware gets better with age. Stains that build up help conduct heat, improving your goodies.

BEST CUTLERY

Using a well-made, sharp knife versus a dull cheapie is like the difference between Michael Phelps's swim stroke and your eight-year-old niece's. A quality blade glides quickly, smoothly, and almost effortlessly through whatever's on your board, making food prep easier, faster, and, for some, downright fun. Don't bother shelling out for a huge set (um, who needs a boning knife?)—you can do just about everything with a few workhorses, only one of which requires a splurge.

Chef's knife. This all-purpose knife will be your kitchen's MVP, so it's worth investing some cash. (Expensive knives perform better.) Look for German brands (such as Wusthof or J. A. Henckels) and Japanese manufacturers (check out Korin.com for the Cadillacs of cutlery). The latter tend to be sharper, with thinner steel, which makes them light but also more delicate—drop one and the tip may crack. German knives are typically sturdier and have more heft, which may help novices feel more comfortable. A standard 8- or 10-inch blade is versatile without being cumbersome, and a good one will cost $130 to $150. Or cut yourself a deal and buy a three-piece starter set with kitchen shears or paring knife and a sharpener. (Skip ceramic knives, which break easily and aren't as versatile.)

Paring knives. Our chef raves about the colorful, all-purpose L'Econome knives, which run a mere $6 a pop at home goods stores and online. Thin, sharp, and easy to handle, you'll use them to slice and peel soft produce such as tomatoes and kiwis, and berries.

Poultry shears. You don't always need a knife to cut and slice. Scissors make for quick, no-hassle prep, such as when you're breaking down cuts of meat or fresh herbs. If you buy a large fillet of salmon, for example, use shears to cut it into single servings. Best part: Kitchen shears are dishwasher-safe.

> Never put your chef's knife in the dishwasher. Water can get between the handle and the steel, creating a fissure that may eventually cause the handle to crack off.

Knife sharpener. If you've never sharpened your knives, now's the time to start. A sharp blade is safer and makes a huge difference in the effort and time you'll need to put into food prep, so sharpen yours every three to six months, or more frequently if you use your knife multiple times per day.

BEST SMALL KITCHEN APPLIANCES

While these aren't essential, they will come in handy, depending on which recipes you make most often.

Coffee grinder. Many Drop 10 recipes call for finely ground coffee beans, and having your own grinder lets you get the right consistency. It can also save you money by turning old-fashioned oats into oat flour (1 cup of oats nets about ¾ cup flour), and you can use one to grind pumpkin seeds and fresh herbs, too. (Be sure to wipe clean after every use.) You don't have to spend a lot—$20 to $30 buys all the power you need.

Immersion blender. This handheld miracle mixes soups, sauces, and dressings, without the fuss of having to pour ingredients and food in and out of a blender. It makes for a quick cleanup, too: Pop off the blade attachment and toss into the dishwasher. And, as with the coffee grinder, save your cash—$30 versions get the job done.

Food processor or mini chopper. A shorter, fatter version of a blender, a food processor finely chops, mixes, and blends more solid foods to make dips and breadings. You can find a large, basic model for about $150, but if you're on a budget, a mini processor (about $40) does everything its daddy can do, though you'll have to work in batches.

BEST UTENSILS AND GADGETS

These basics belong in every kitchen—even take-out queens need at least a few things in their drawers! They'll make prep for the Drop 10 recipes a breeze.

Box grater. Not only for cheese, stand-up box graters rip through apples, sweet potatoes, carrots, and other produce that you'll slip into muffins and quick breads, sauces, soups, salads, and other dishes.

Cutting boards. You need two—one for meat, poultry, and fish and one for produce to avoid contaminating your fruit and veggies with bacteria that can live on raw proteins. Choose any material you like except glass, which tortures knives (and your ears for the sound it makes). You may prefer plastic, anyway; it doesn't need to be treated with mineral oil like wood and bamboo, and it's dishwasher-safe.

Citrus squeezer or reamer. Your hands and fingers can only do so much! These little tools help you squeeze the most out of every lemon and lime.

Microplane zester. This tool looks like a long, thin grater and is useful for not only citrus fruits but also garlic, nutmeg, and hard cheeses, such as Parmesan.

Measuring cups and spoons. You need these for obvious reasons, but measuring cups with handles (they look like ladles) can double as serving utensils, helping you control portion sizes.

Pepper mill. You can't do much with those fresh peppercorns unless you've got something to grind them!

Plastic storage containers. Go for the thin bargain varieties to keep cut fruit and veggies, sandwiches, salads, and other cold food and leftovers fresh. Look for brands such as Ziploc and Glad, which are free of BPA, a chemical found in some plastic that may potentially have health effects.

Glass storage containers. Along with your stash of plastic, get a set of glass containers to use for hot food. With glass, you can spoon piping-hot meals directly in without worrying about plastic melting or leaching into your lunch and imparting a toxic taste. (Let it cool down before sealing and storing.) Glass is also safer for microwave reheating and won't stain.

Rubber spatulas. Pick up a large and mini size to scrape every last bit of muffin mix, sauce, dip, and the like out of bowls, pots, and your food processor. The tiny spatulas also help you get your money's worth out of a jar of salsa or mayo.

Salad spinner. This tool helps you wash and dry greens and other veggies in a flash. Opt for one with a nice-looking outer bowl, which can double as a serving dish for cold items.

Tongs. Not only for grilling, tongs toss salads, serve up pasta, and come in handy for countless other tasks. No need to pony up for a fancy pair—inexpensive metal ones are light and easy to use.

Wooden spoons. Sturdy and inexpensive. Opt for several different sizes. Unlike plastic, wood won't melt if you set it against a hot pan, nor bend when stirring batter.

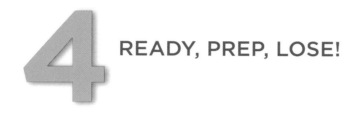

4 READY, PREP, LOSE!

NOW THAT YOU'VE PRIMED YOUR KITCHEN, STOCKED UP ON essentials, and are familiar with the Drop 10 superfoods, it's time to get cooking! Even if you've never so much as microwaved popcorn, you can begin churning out scrumptious dishes today.

You could turn straight to the recipes on page 53, but it's worth your while to read this chapter first. Think of it as Drop 10 grad school, where you'll learn insider tips for planning, prep, and cooking. Don't let the idea of school throw you—the tutorials are all quick and easy. Check out this mini syllabus, then dig into your first lesson.

Menu planning. You'll find simple ways to chart out meals to help you shed fat.

Knife skills. Knowing how to handle a blade slashes prep time.

Cooking tips. These hints offer pearls of prepping wisdom for superfoods (like quinoa) that you may want to make ahead of time.

MEAL PLANNING MADE SIMPLE

Spontaneity is a wonderful thing when you're on vacation, but for your diet, it's a recipe for disaster. Consider those times you've opened the fridge or pantry after a long day, and, upon seeing a random mishmash of cans, produce, and leftovers, shut the door and opened a take-out menu instead. Or perhaps you opt for a blah frozen dinner, only to find yourself scraping the bottom of a carton of ice cream two hours later.

Whether your goal is to lose fat, boost your health, or simply cook more at home, you are more likely to succeed if you plot your week's meals and shop ahead of time. Knowing exactly which tasty, fat-fighting meal you'll make for dinner or pack for lunch before your stomach starts growling—and having everything you need on hand—puts pound melting on autopilot. In fact, planning ahead helps you make more rational, healthier decisions about food, suggests a study from Harvard University. You'll also be more likely to skirt the inner turmoil that comes with deciding between what you *should* do to reach your goals (go to the grocery store, fire up the stove) versus what's easiest in the moment (drive-through burgers or pizza delivery). And if that's not enough to convince you to plan ahead, try this: The average woman tosses out nearly $1,000 worth of food per year. Writing up a weekly menu and buying only what you need guarantees your grocery budget feeds only you and your family, not your trash bin.

Sure, you'll have to front a little time, but it's less of a hassle than you might think and beats the alternative—gaining extra pounds. Use the easy guide here to map out a week's worth of healthy, speedy meals.

1. **Pick your day.** Decide when it's most convenient to choose your menu and shop. If you work a nine-to-five, try a weekend morning and make this time a pleasure: Pour a cup of coffee (a superfood!), play music, and even put your feet up while you make your list.

2. **Scan your schedule.** Think of each day's breakfast, lunch, dinner, and snack as a slot to fill. If you've got a work dinner on Tuesday, a lunch meeting on Thursday, and girls' night out on Saturday, that leaves the rest of your slots open to fill with dishes that sound good to you. Jot them directly into your calendar or use a blank one you designate for meals only and tack up in the kitchen.

3. **Aim for diversity.** The more different superfoods you eat, the better your odds of slimming success, so branch out. Try for at least two fish meals per week and sprinkle in a few vegetarian options, as well. Also, don't forget healthy, grab-and-go snacks such as fresh fruit, veggies, nuts, and those in chapter 7. And of course, if you're following the full Drop 10 diet plan, think about how you want to spend your happy calories.

4. Plan for leftovers. Depending on how many people you cook for, Monday night's meat loaf could morph into a brown-bag sandwich for Tuesday's lunch. If you feed a whole houseful, double down on a few recipes so you'll have extra portions to eat later. Just be sure to pack away the extra helpings before you sit down to eat so you aren't tempted to gobble up tomorrow's lunch.

5. Make your list. Take a quick inventory of what you've already got, then jot down what you need to buy for the week's recipes. To speed your shopping, organize your list according to where foods are in the store—group together meats and seafood, fruits and veggies, milk and cheese, so on.

6. Check it twice. Be sure you've marked everything you need, because if you forget something, it's often best to truly forget it. Quick trips for one or two ingredients can lead to impulse purchases that can hurt you both on the scale and in the wallet.

7. Break it down. When you get home from shopping, chop veggies for recipes, salads, and sides, wash and slice fruit so it's ready to eat, portion out large packages and snacks into smaller servings, marinate or freeze meats and seafood, and do anything else you can to shorten up prep time in the days ahead. Storing everything in clear glass containers looks appealing and encourages you to munch on the healthy stuff. Once everything is packed away, kick back and admire your handiwork, knowing that soon you'll be admiring your pound-peeling success in the mirror, too.

CHOP, SLICE, AND DICE IN SECONDS

If you think chopping veggies, fruit, and herbs is tedious or even a literal pain—nothing hurts like accidentally carving up a finger (yeouch!)—chances are, you're doing it wrong. We tend to enjoy doing what we're good at, and if prepping a salad leaves your counter resembling a produce crime scene strewn with mangled veggies, we don't blame you for fleeing the kitchen.

The good news is you don't have to enroll in Le Cordon Bleu to learn how to handle a knife as proficiently as you do your smartphone. Even better, learning basic knife skills can change the way you feel about cooking. Not only will you have more fun and cut prep time, you'll build valuable kitchen confidence. That can give you the courage to experiment with new flavors and unique foods, which is exactly what eating is all about. Now don your apron, grab your knife, and let's do this. Chop, chop!

1. GET A GRIP

Grab the handle near where it meets the blade and curl your last three fingers around it. Then place your pointer and thumb on opposite sides of the blade. Most people hold the handle too far back and plop their index finger on top, but gripping both sides of the steel gives you more control, especially since you'll do the majority of your chopping on the part of the blade close to the handle.

2. GO THROUGH THE MOTIONS

When making your first cut into large fruits, veggies, and other foods, place the tip of the blade on the food, then push down and forward in one fluid move. To julienne veggies, or chop or dice small or long items (green onions, carrots, celery), use the portion of the blade from the midpoint to the heel (the part closest to the handle). Keep the tip on the cutting board and use the same motion described above—but after pushing the knife down and forward, lift the handle to move it back and up, then repeat, almost like a sawing motion. (The tip should stay in contact with your cutting board.) As you chop, keep your knife in place and "feed" the food into it as if on a slow-moving conveyer belt. Don't stress if you don't get the technique down the first few times or aren't going as quickly as TV chefs do—the more you practice, the better and faster you'll become.

3. DEFEND YOUR DIGITS

Wondering what to do with your other hand, the one that directs food into the blade? Rather than holding food with the pads of your fingertips—which serves them up like a neck for the guillotine—curl each finger as if making a claw. Secure and move food with the tops of your fingers, which pushes your knuckles out; the area between your first and second knuckle should be parallel to the side of the blade. And watch that pinkie! It naturally wants to relax, so if you see it starting to hang loose, rein it in. Same goes for your thumb.

4. ADAPT YOUR APPROACH

You'll use this basic technique and sawing motion all the time to slice, dice, and chop, but certain foods require a little windup first:

Large, rounded fruit and veggies. Whether you're dicing onions, slicing sweet potato fries, or chopping an apple, always cut the food in half first and lay the flat side down to create a still, steady piece for you to work on. For foods such as onions and sweet potatoes, you may want to make additional cuts to square off the edges to make a brick. Then simply cut into long strips. In a dicey situation? When making your lengthwise cuts, leave about ½ inch at the end of your brick intact. Make your horizontal cuts, then vertical, so you end up with tidy, tiny cubes.

Bell peppers and jalapeños. Cut off both ends and stand the pepper upright on your cutting board. Make a single slice, top to bottom, and unroll. With your blade parallel

---

TAKE ON THE TOUGHIES

Not all fruits and veggies are so straightforward to prep. (Hello, artichokes!) Use these simple tips to make quick work of the trickier Drop 10 superfoods.

Artichokes. In recipes, you'll use only the hearts; buy them frozen to save yourself money and time. But for snacking, you can't beat a fresh choke. To turn the prickly globes into something you actually want to eat, cut off the stem and about ½ inch off the top. Steam in a steamer basket for about forty-five minutes or microwave in half an inch of water for six to eight minutes. Once tender, pluck off the petals one by one, scraping the base of each between your teeth to eat the soft inside. Cut the remaining part in half, then scoop out and eat the heart.

Avocado. Using a small chef's knife, carefully slice through the fruit lengthwise around the seed; twist the halves and pull apart. Carefully pop out the seed with the tip of your knife, then use a spoon to scoop out the flesh in one piece.

Kale. Each large kale leaf sports a rigid stem and thick, bitter-tasting spine you'll want to discard. After rinsing, lay each leaf flat and slice on either side of the spine. Then stack a few leaves and use your basic knife technique to cut into long ribbons or pieces. If you aren't concerned about neat edges (for instance, when you're prepping kale for a smoothie), skip the knife and simply tear the leaves from the spine and into smaller pieces.

Pomegranate. Ever tried cutting a pomegranate like an orange? It's not pretty—renegade spurts of juice can rack up a hefty dry-cleaning bill! A better way: Cut off the fruit's spiky crown and make four shallow cuts from top to base. Submerge the fruit in a bowl of water to avoid sprays as you break it apart along the cuts. Use your fingers to gently pull off the juicy arils and separate them from their white pith.

to the board, gently slice off the raised white veins and seedy core. Then use the basic chopping technique above to cut into four sections. Keeping the skin side down, make two stacks of two and slice. To dice, turn strips 90 degrees and cut again. Then dice the top and bottom you previously sliced off.

Thick-skinned fruit. To get at the sweet flesh of a pineapple, mango, or other produce, start by slicing off the top and bottom, then standing the fruit upright on your cutting board. Using your chef's knife, a paring knife (for smaller fruits), or an inexpensive serrated bread knife, slowly cut along the curve of the fruit, removing the rind in sections. Next, cut the fruit into quarters, and slice away any core. Place the fruit on a flat side to slice or dice to your desired size.

Leafy herbs. Don't bother picking the leaves off cilantro—the stems are just as flavorful. Lay the bunch flat and cut off and discard the long, leafless bottom portion of the stem. Keeping the tip of your blade on the cutting board, chop the herb, using the section of the knife from center to heel. Don't feed it into the blade; instead, pivot it to chop, placing your usual feeder hand on top of the blade to direct and stabilize it. For basil, mint, parsley, and rosemary, do pick off leaves, then chop, using the same pivot motion.

COOKING TIPS FROM THE DROP 10 TEST KITCHEN

Most of the Drop 10 superfoods require nothing more than chopping or measuring before they're incorporated into a recipe. A select few, however, may need a smidge more attention before they're ready for the skillet or plate. Our chef treated us to her insider tricks for these special cases.

PREP TIPS FOR PRODUCE

Frozen fruit and veggies. Place your pick in a bowl and let sit on the counter. Most fruits and veggies thaw in less than fifteen minutes, but chopping or running water over them can speed things up.

Sweet potatoes. For recipes that call for pre-cooked potatoes, you can always use canned, but fresh baked spuds are easy to use and stay fresh up to four days in the fridge or up to about six months in the freezer. Regardless of the cooking methods you use, always wash your sweet potato and poke holes in the skin with a fork first. To bake, loosely wrap each potato in aluminum foil; place on a baking sheet and cook at 350°F for an hour. Or cut potatoes in half to trim cooking time to about forty-five minutes.

The foil makes for quick cleanup, since natural sugars in your spud can turn to syrup and be a nightmare to remove. Your potato is done when it is very soft—give it a squeeze or a poke with a fork to check. To microwave, wrap each whole spud in a paper towel and set inside the microwave; cook on high five to six minutes.

PREP TIPS FOR GRAINS AND LEGUMES

Lentils and quinoa are perfect make-ahead foods and stay fresh for about a week in the fridge; the same for popcorn, as long as you store it in an airtight bag in the pantry. Why not make a big batch of each this Sunday? With pasta, you're best off making it fresh, although leftovers will keep for about a week in the fridge.

Lentils. One of the biggest mistakes people make is overcooking these fiber-rich belly flatteners. They hold their shape and taste best when cooked slightly al dente, so they're firm, almost like brown rice. Try it: Bring a few cups of water to a boil while you rinse the lentils and pick out any debris. Add the lentils to the boiling water and reduce the heat to low. Simmer red lentils about fifteen minutes, brown and green for twenty to twenty-five minutes. Drain.

Popcorn. If you can find plain microwave corn (topping-free, low-fat, low-sodium), you can use that. But loose kernels are a lot cheaper (around 25 cents less per ounce) and don't require much more effort to pop with one of these methods:

- **AIR POPPING.** A no-fuss machine, which you can buy for about $30, yields a super-skinny snack that's 31 calories per cup.
- **MICROWAVE AIR POPPING.** If you don't want to pony up for the machine, you can turn your microwave into an air popper. Place ¼ cup kernels in a paper bag, fold over the top a few times so the bag stays closed but not sealed tight, and cook on high two to three minutes.
- **STOVETOP.** This method requires oil, which bumps up your calorie count to 55 per cup, but also boosts flavor. Heat a large skillet or heavy pot on high; pour in 1 teaspoon canola oil for every ¾ cup kernels. Cover and cook two to three minutes, or until the popping subsides. Don't use olive oil—the high heat can cause it to smoke and burn, leaving you with charred corn.

Quinoa. Adding this grain to baked goods, such as the Breakfast Banana Bread on page 90, adds mouthwatering moistness. You must cook it first, however. The method is identical to that for rice, so use a rice cooker if you've got one; go with the same ratio of water to quinoa as you would for white rice. Or prepare quinoa on the stove. After rinsing to remove the grain's bitter coating, combine 2 cups water for every cup quinoa and bring to a boil. Reduce the heat, cover, and simmer about fifteen minutes or until all the water is absorbed and you see white "tails" spiraling out of each grain.

Whole-grain pasta. Different grains and grain blends require slightly different cooking times, so always follow the directions on the box. You may want to cook whole-wheat noodles a minute or two longer than you would white pasta, to help soften their texture. But taste-test often to avoid crossing over from pleasantly chewy to gummy. Also, be careful not to overcook pasta made with quinoa and brown rice. Even an extra minute can turn these noodles mushy.

PREP TIPS FOR STEAK, FISH, AND EGGS

Always pat-dry your meat and fish with a paper towel before cooking. Doing so will give you a better sear and prevent the protein from steam-cooking.

Steak. You'll notice that many of the recipes suggest searing steak first; this adds flavor by breaking down proteins on the surface of beef, unlocking its full, rich taste. To seal in the juice, give it a rest: After grilling, searing, or roasting, allow your meat to sit on a clean plate for a few minutes before slicing. Meat fibers are shaped like an accordion—they open when exposed to heat and contract as they cool. Cutting into a hot steak too soon, before the juices have had a chance to seep back into the open fibers, can cause all that moisture to flood out onto your cutting board.

Salmon. Searing fish also enhances flavor, plus gives it a more beautiful, appetizing look. If you buy your fish with the skin, it's okay to keep it on during cooking. Sear skin-side up first, then flip, giving that side a few extra minutes to cook. Once you're done, the skin should come off easily. Also keep in mind that wild salmon cooks more quickly than farm-raised, since it's typically leaner.

Eggs. It's been said that the mark of a great chef is a perfectly cooked egg. Try these no-fail methods:

- SUNNY-SIDE UP. Heat a skillet over high heat. Remove the skillet from the heat, mist with cooking spray, and return to the stove. Reduce the heat to medium. (Heat that's either too high or too low may cause eggs to stick to the pan.) Crack your egg in the center and cook for 3 to 4 minutes, or until the whites are firm but the yolk is still runny.
- HARD-BOILED. Submerge eggs in cool water in a saucepan and bring to a boil. Once boiling, immediately cover the pan, turn off the heat, and let sit for 15 min-

utes. This technique results in fluffier yolks with no green discoloration, as can occur if you drop eggs into boiling water.

For recipes that call for coffee grounds, be sure to set your grinder on the finest setting (sometimes called Turkish grind). Your grounds should be about the consistency of flour. For dishes that use brewed coffee, fire up your coffeemaker or opt for an inexpensive cup-top brewer, such as those from Melitta.

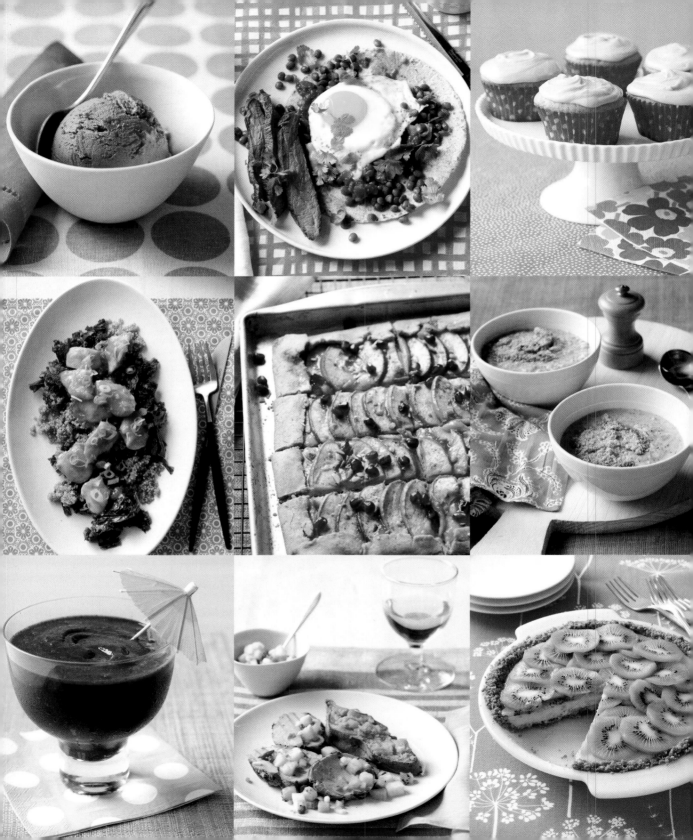

THE
RECIPES

RECIPE KEY

These icons let you quickly identify the dishes that best fit your lifestyle and needs.

EAT ON THE GO
Tasty bites for times you have to dine as you dash.

FAST (10 MINUTES, MAX)
Time not on your side? These recipes are!

FREEZER-READY
These are the Drop 10 healthier versions of frozen meals.

GREAT FOR GUESTS
Serve these and let the compliments roll in!

KID-FRIENDLY
Even your pickiest critics will clean their plate.

MAKE-AHEAD
Prep 'em and forget 'em until it's time to eat.

NO-COOK
Give your stove, oven, and microwave the day off.

VEGETARIAN
No meat or fish, but you may find eggs and dairy.*

* Some recipes with the vegetarian icon contain Parmesan, which is sometimes made with rennet derived from animals. If you're vegetarian, look for brands that specifically say they are vegetarian on the label; they're likely made with microbial rennet or plant-based rennet.

5 EASY, ENERGIZING BREAKFASTS

AHHH, MORNING: A QUIET TIME TO RELAX OVER COFFEE AND the paper before your day shifts into gear. Yeah, right! Some days it's a miracle you manage to get dressed, much less make and eat a healthy breakfast. So we understand why you may skip it or grab a big latte or a doughnut instead.

But if there's anything in your current routine worth reevaluating, it's your morning meal. Aside from being a pleasurable way to start your day, eating in the a.m. may be a key weight management strategy. Studies link skipping breakfast with being overweight or obese—in fact, research published in the *American Journal of Epidemiology* pegged the increased risk of obesity as four and a half times greater! Filling up on healthy eats first thing may help tame hunger-stimulating insulin into the afternoon.

Most of the breakfasts in this chapter check in at about 350 calories, despite plate-filling portions. (A few are a little higher or lower, to allow for flexibility in your menu planning.) They also pack plenty of satiating, flab-fighting protein, fiber, and healthy fats to keep your belly full and cravings silent without increasing your day's calorie tally. What you will increase by eating these dishes: *yums* and *mmms*.

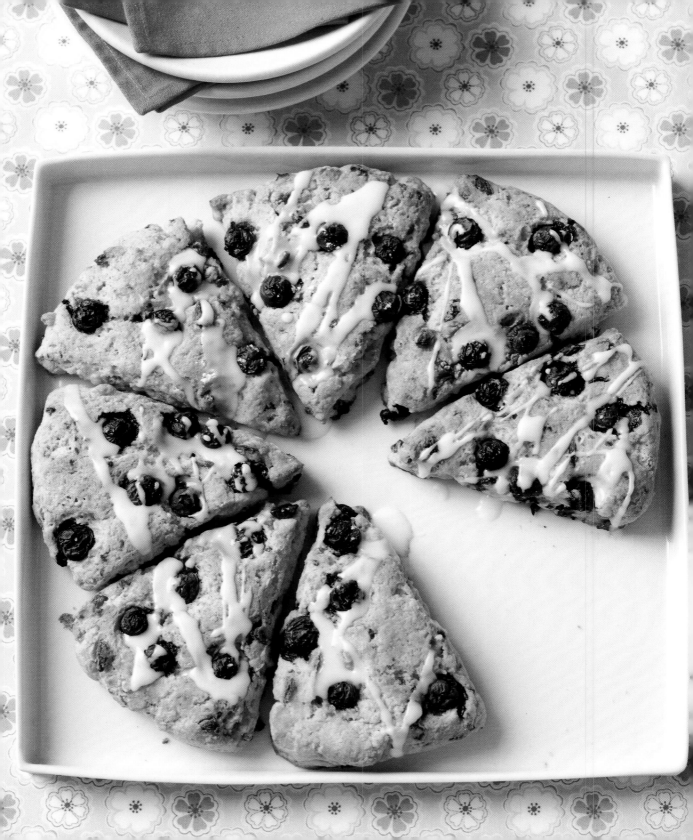

GLAZED BLUEBERRY GOJI SCONES

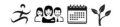

Makes 8 scones • SUPERFOODS: Blueberries, Cherries, Goji Berries, Oats, Yogurt

Coffee shop scones can weigh in at nearly 500 calories a pop. The Drop 10 version matches them in size and devour-ability, but with fewer than 250 calories each.

Olive oil cooking spray
1 ½ cups oat flour
½ cup all-purpose flour, plus extra
    to flour hands
¼ cup sugar
1 tablespoon baking powder

5 tablespoons unsalted butter,
    cold, cut into chunks
6 tablespoons goji berries
¼ cup dried cherries
1 cup low-fat plain Greek yogurt
1 cup fresh or frozen blueberries,
    thawed

LEMON GLAZE:

2 tablespoons powdered sugar,
    sifted
2 tablespoons plain, low-fat Greek
    yogurt

1 lemon, zested and juiced (about
    ¼ cup juice)

Heat the oven to 400°F. Coat a large baking sheet with cooking spray.

In a food processor, pulse together the flours, sugar, and baking powder. Add the butter and pulse eight times, until the butter creates small crumbs in the flour.

Add the goji berries, cherries, and yogurt. Pulse until just combined. Flour hands. Transfer the dough onto the cooking sheet and pat into an 8-inch round disk. Press the blueberries over the top and cut the disk into eight equal wedges, spacing them 1 inch apart.

Bake 15 to 20 minutes, until the tops brown. Cool on the baking sheet for 10 minutes before glazing.

PREPARE THE GLAZE:

In a small bowl, place the powdered sugar and yogurt and whisk until smooth. Add the juice and zest and whisk again until well combined. Spoon over the scones and serve.

(1 GLAZED SCONE) 244 CALORIES, 7 G PROTEIN, 9 G FAT (5 G SATURATED), 36 G CARBOHYDRATES, 4 G FIBER, 128 MG SODIUM

BEEFY BREAKFAST BURRITO

SERVES 1 • SUPERFOODS: Eggs, Steak, Yogurt

A gift for your fat-fighting efforts, this hearty meal wraps up loads of hunger-squashing protein and fiber in a tasty, grab-and-go package. Need to make a quick exit in the morning? Roll one up the night before and store it in the fridge, and you can kiss those cardboardy frozen burritos good-bye.

1 8-inch whole-wheat wrap

Nonstick cooking spray

2 ounces raw flank steak (or $^3/_4$ packed cup of leftover
   Coffee Chili-Rubbed Flank Steak, page 135)

$^1/_8$ teaspoon salt

1 egg

1 cup baby spinach, finely chopped

$^1/_4$ cup plain, low-fat yogurt

Heat the oven to 200°F. Place the wrap in the oven. Heat a small skillet over high heat. Remove the skillet from the heat and coat with cooking spray. Return the skillet to the

> ### EGGS-CELLENT CHOICE
> Fueling up on eggs in the morning helps you eat less all day, ultimately trimming your weight and waist.

heat. Sprinkle the steak with the salt and place it in the skillet. Reduce the heat to medium and cook the steak, turning once, about 12 minutes. (Beef should be medium-rare.) Remove from the skillet and transfer to a cutting board.

In a small bowl, place the egg, spinach, and yogurt and whisk to combine. Heat another small skillet over medium heat. Remove the skillet from the heat and coat with cooking spray. Return the skillet to heat. Add the egg mixture and cook about 1 minute, stirring once or twice, until soft curds form. Remove from the heat. Slice the steak. Remove the wrap from the oven and layer with the cooked egg mixture and the steak. Roll up and serve immediately, or wrap in aluminum foil to go.

(1 BURRITO) 298 CALORIES, 31 G PROTEIN, 13 G FAT (4 G SATURATED), 26 G CARBOHYDRATES, 14 G FIBER, 805 MG SODIUM

CHEF'S NOTE:
Using leftover beef? Skip the salt.

JELLY DOUGHNUT SMOOTHIE

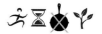

SERVES 1 • SUPERFOODS: Blueberries, Coffee, Peanuts, Yogurt

The berries satisfy your sweet tooth, and the combo of peanuts, coffee, and a hint of sugar trick your taste buds into thinking, *Mmm, fried dough*. The metabolism boost and fat-fighting fiber you can score with every sip are icing on the cake.

1 1/2 cups fresh or frozen blueberries

1 cup plain low-fat yogurt

2 tablespoons chopped unsalted, dry-roasted peanuts

1/4 cup brewed coffee

4 ice cubes

1 tablespoon granulated sugar

Place all ingredients in a blender, and blend until smooth. Serve immediately.

(2 CUPS) 401 CALORIES, 16 G PROTEIN, 12 G FAT (4 G SATURATED), 61 G CARBOHYDRATES, 11 G FIBER, 242 MG SODIUM

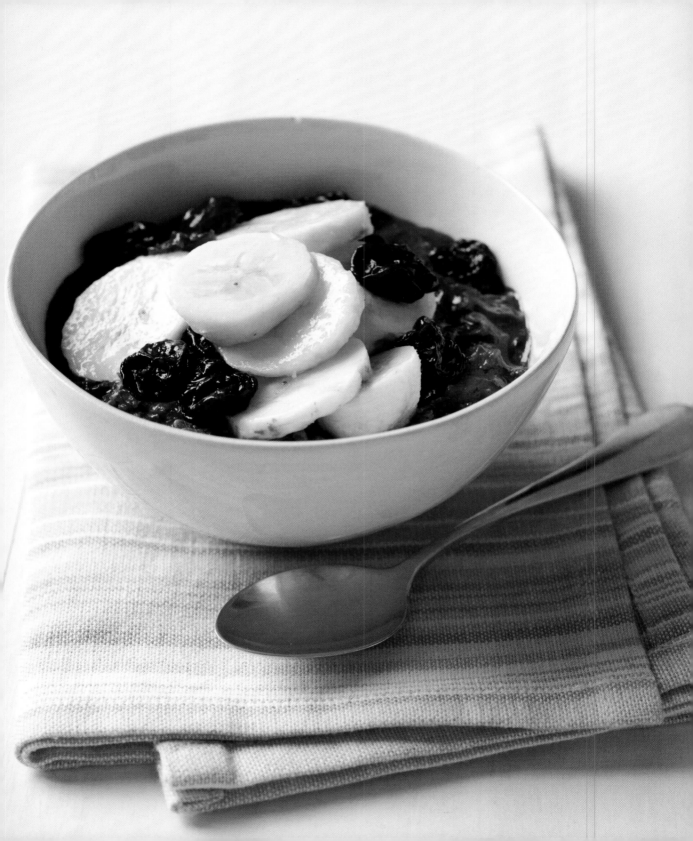

COCOA OATMEAL

SERVES 1 • SUPERFOODS: Cherries, Coffee, Dark Chocolate, Oats

Hot cereal can be a snooze, but you'll want to jump out of bed for this delicious mix of dried cherries, rich chocolate, and coffee in warm, creamy oats. Think of it as your grown-up, slimmed-down version of childhood cocoa cereal.

3/4 cup skim milk

1/2 cup brewed coffee

1/2 cup old-fashioned oats

1 tablespoon unsweetened cocoa powder

1 tablespoon brown sugar

2 tablespoons dried cherries

1/2 ripe banana, sliced

Place the skim milk and coffee in a small saucepan. Bring to a simmer over medium heat. Add the oats and cocoa powder; stir well. Reduce the heat to low and cook until the oats are soft and a loose porridge begins to form, 4 to 5 minutes. Remove from the heat, add the brown sugar, and stir well. Pour into a bowl. Top with cherries and banana and serve.

362 CALORIES, 13 G PROTEIN, 4 G FAT (1 G SATURATED), 76 G CARBOHYDRATES, 8 G FIBER, 85 MG SODIUM

CHEF'S NOTE:
Brewing coffee to sip? Make a few extra cups. Store cooled coffee in a clean jar in the fridge for up to 1 week to use in recipes like this one.

LEMON BLUEBERRY CRUNCH

SERVES 4 • SUPERFOODS: Blueberries, Eggs, Goji Berries, Oats, Olive Oil, Peanuts, Pumpkin Seeds, Quinoa, Yogurt

Most yogurt parfaits leave you wondering, *Is that it*? You'll need a bigger cup for this one! The usual sugary granola swaps out for a satisfying mix of pound-shedding protein, belly-flattening fiber, and healthy, filling fats, all sweetened with a touch of maple syrup. Plump blueberries and creamy yogurt round out the layers.

1/4 cup maple syrup	2 tablespoons goji berries
1 egg white	1/4 teaspoon ground cinnamon
2 teaspoons olive oil	2 cups plain low-fat Greek yogurt
1 cup old-fashioned oats	1/2 lemon, zested and juiced
1/2 cup cooked quinoa	3 tablespoons powdered sugar
2 tablespoons pumpkin seeds	2 cups blueberries
2 tablespoons peanuts	

Heat the oven to 250°F. Place the maple syrup, egg white, and olive oil in a medium bowl. Stir well. Add the oats, quinoa, pumpkin seeds, peanuts, goji berries, and cinnamon, and toss well to coat. Transfer to two ungreased baking sheets and spread out into a thin layer. Bake 40 to 45 minutes, until crisp. Cool on the baking sheets.

> ### SWEET TALK
>
> When you're buying maple syrup, choose a bottle that lists only one ingredient: maple syrup. Some brands contain very little of the actual tree sap and instead use high-fructose corn syrup and other added sugars and artificial flavors.

Place the yogurt, lemon zest and juice, and powdered sugar in a small bowl. Mix until well combined. Place 1/2 cup blueberries in each of four ramekins or parfait cups. Top each with an equal amount of the yogurt blend. Divide the oat-quinoa mixture evenly over each and serve immediately.

THE DISH (1 1/2 CUPS) 374 CALORIES, 18 G PROTEIN, 11 G FAT (32 G SATURATED), 58 G CARBOHYDRATES, 5 G FIBER, 115 MG SODIUM

CHEF'S NOTE:
The crunchy baked layer of this parfait doubles as a stick-to-your-ribs hot cereal. Serve with 1/2 cup skim milk and a piece of fresh fruit.

CHOCOLATE CHUNK AND CHERRY PANCAKES

SERVES 6 (makes 18 pancakes) • SUPERFOODS: Cherries, Dark Chocolate, Eggs, Goji Berries, Oats, Olive Oil

Thought loaded pancakes were a diet no-no? No, no, not on Drop 10! Serve these haute cakes, stacked with fiber, at your next brunch and your guests will marvel only at their deliciousness—until, of course, you reveal their awe-inspiring calorie count.

1 1/2 cups oat flour

1 cup whole-wheat flour

2 teaspoons baking powder

1 teaspoon baking soda

2 cups skim milk

2 eggs

1 tablespoon brown sugar

1 tablespoon light olive oil

1/2 teaspoon vanilla extract

1/2 cup 70% cacao chocolate chunks (break up a bar)

2 tablespoons dried cherries, chopped

2 tablespoons goji berries

Nonstick cooking spray

In a large bowl, mix together the flours, baking powder, and baking soda. Set aside.

In a medium bowl, whisk together the milk, eggs, brown sugar, olive oil, and vanilla extract. Pour into the flour mixture and add the chocolate, cherries, and goji berries. Whisk until a loose batter forms; do not overmix (a few lumps are fine). The batter will be looser than a traditional pancake batter, but will firm as it cooks.

Heat a large skillet over medium-high heat. Remove the skillet from the heat, coat with cooking spray, and return to the stove.

Using a 1/4-cup measure, drop four dollops of batter into the skillet, spacing the pancakes 1 inch apart. Reduce the heat to medium and cook 4 to 5 minutes, until the edges firm and tiny bubbles form over the surface of the pancakes. Flip and cook 2 minutes or until the pancakes are firm to the touch and cooked through. Repeat to make 18 cakes.

(3 PANCAKES) 340 CALORIES, 12 G PROTEIN, 11 G FAT (4 G SATURATED), 54 G CARBOHYDRATES, 7 G FIBER, 405 MG SODIUM

APPLE PARMESAN FRITTERS

SERVES 4 (makes 16 cakes total) • SUPERFOODS: Apples, Eggs, Olive Oil, Parmesan, Quinoa, Yogurt

Satisfyingly sweet and savory, these pan-fried fritters aren't the calorie bombs you'd expect, thanks to the fiber-filled apples and protein-heavy quinoa and yogurt, which lend a firm, hearty texture sans the extra grease.

1 cup soft white whole-wheat flour (such as King Arthur) or whole-wheat pastry flour
$\frac{1}{2}$ cup grated Parmesan
1 teaspoon granulated sugar
$\frac{1}{4}$ teaspoon baking powder
$\frac{1}{4}$ teaspoon salt
$\frac{1}{4}$ teaspoon freshly ground black pepper
2 apples, such as Gala or Golden Delicious, grated (about 1 $\frac{1}{4}$ cups)

$\frac{1}{2}$ cup cooked quinoa, room temperature or chilled
$\frac{1}{2}$ cup plain, low-fat Greek yogurt
2 eggs, lightly beaten
2 scallions, thinly sliced (green and white parts), divided
8 teaspoons olive oil, divided

In a large bowl, mix together the flour, Parmesan, sugar, baking powder, salt, and black pepper. Make a well in the center of the mixture and add the grated apple, quinoa, yogurt, eggs, and half the scallions. Using a wooden spoon, stir the contents in the well ten to fifteen times, gradually incorporating the flour mixture to create a batter. Do not overmix.

Heat a large skillet over medium-high heat. Add 2 teaspoons of the olive oil and tilt the pan to coat. Drop a scant $\frac{1}{4}$ cup of the batter into the pan four times, spacing the fritters about an inch apart. Cook each until they are golden and starting to brown at the edges, 3 to 4 minutes. Flip and cook 2 minutes, until the cakes are golden and cooked through. Transfer to a plate. Coat the pan with 2 teaspoons of olive oil and repeat the process; continue until you have made sixteen cakes. Garnish with the remaining scallions. Top with a dollop of yogurt, if desired.

(4 FRITTERS) 362 CALORIES, 16 G PROTEIN, 15 G FAT (4 G SATURATED), 43 G CARBOHYDRATES, 6 G FIBER, 374 MG SODIUM

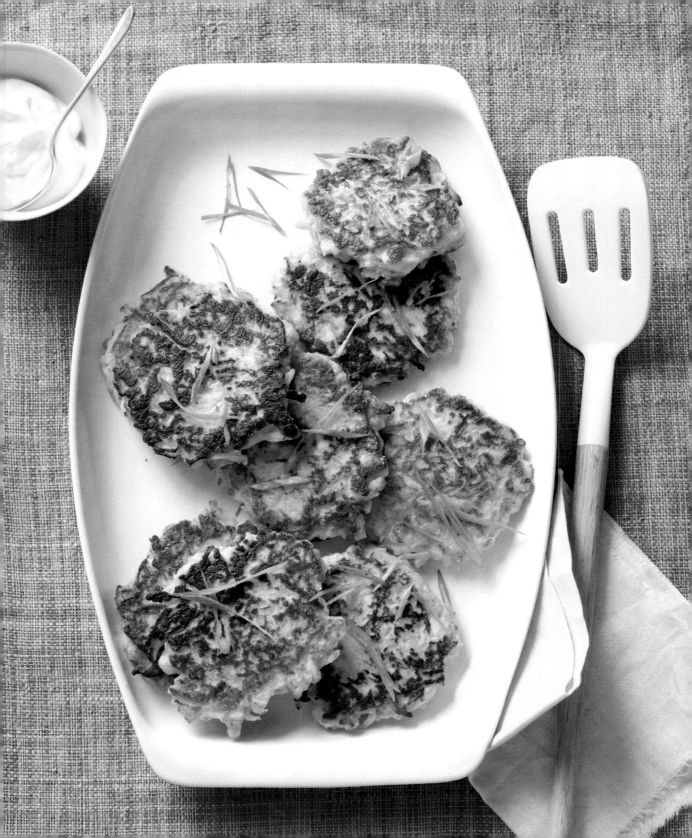

MUSHROOM FONTINA OMELET

SERVES 4 • SUPERFOODS: Eggs, Mushrooms, Olive Oil, Yogurt

The omelet gets a superfood makeover! Greek yogurt replaces milk, nearly doubling the satiating protein while maintaining a light, fluffy texture.

1 tablespoon olive oil
10 ounces mushrooms, such as
    cremini or white button, sliced
    (about 4 cups)
1/2 cup chopped red onion
1 teaspoon chopped fresh
    rosemary
1/4 teaspoon salt

1/4 teaspoon crushed red pepper
    (optional)
8 eggs
1/2 cup plain low-fat Greek yogurt
1/4 cup fresh basil leaves, chopped
Nonstick cooking spray
1/2 cup grated Fontina cheese

Heat a large skillet over medium heat. Add the olive oil, mushrooms, onion, rosemary, salt, and crushed red pepper (if desired). Cook 5 to 6 minutes, stirring often, until the mushrooms release their liquid and shrink by half. Turn off the heat and set aside.

> **TABLE FOR 1?**
>
> Make a single-serving omelet using 2 eggs, 1/8 cup each Greek yogurt, cheese, and onion, and 2 1/2 ounces mushrooms (about 1 cup).

Place the eggs, yogurt, and basil in a large bowl. Whisk well. Heat another large skillet over high heat. Remove the skillet from the burner and coat with cooking spray. Return the skillet to the stove. Reduce the heat to medium and add the egg mixture. As it cooks, pull the cooked edges of the eggs back toward the center of the pan and tilt the pan to allow some of the uncooked mixture to settle around the edge. Repeat two or three times until you have a thicker center, and the eggs are almost cooked through.

Spoon the mushrooms over half the egg and top it with the Fontina. Cover, reduce the heat to low, and cook 1 minute. Tip the pan forward and flip the empty side of the omelet over the half with the mushrooms. Cover to allow the cheese to melt, 30 seconds. Remove from the heat, cut into four wedges, and serve immediately.

288 CALORIES, 23 G PROTEIN, 19 G FAT (7 G SATURATED), 6 G CARBOHYDRATES, 2 G FIBER, 460 MG SODIUM

LEMON CREPES WITH CHERRY-RICOTTA FILLING

SERVES 4 • SUPERFOODS: Cherries, Eggs, Oats, Olive Oil, Yogurt

Crepes typically ooze fat like the French ooze sex appeal, but you can say *bonjour* to two (yes, two!) of these skinny delights. Skim milk, part-skim ricotta, and low-fat Greek yogurt cut the saturated fat and calories but deliver plenty of calcium (nearly half your day's worth) to help your body burn fat more efficiently.

2 cups skim milk

1 cup whole-wheat pastry flour or soft whole-wheat flour

$1/2$ cup oat flour

2 tablespoons golden or plain ground flax

2 eggs

2 tablespoons sugar

1 tablespoon light olive oil

$1/4$ teaspoon salt

Nonstick cooking spray

1 cup part-skim ricotta cheese

1 cup fresh or frozen cherries, chopped

$1/2$ cup plain, low-fat Greek yogurt

$1/4$ cup powdered sugar

2 teaspoons lemon zest

Place the milk, flours, flax, eggs, granulated sugar, olive oil, and salt in a blender. Process until smooth. Refrigerate, covered, for 1 hour.

Heat a griddle or a crepe pan over medium heat. Coat with cooking spray. (If you're using a pan, remove it from the heat, spray, and return to the heat). Spoon out $1/4$ cup of the batter onto the griddle and spread it out with a small spatula; or, if you're using a crepe pan, tilt it until the bottom is totally covered with batter. Cook 2 to 3 minutes, until the crepe begins to brown around the edges and dry out on top. Flip and cook 1 minute, until the crepe is no longer wet in the center. Remove the crepe from the heat and set it aside on a plate. Repeat with the remaining batter to make eight crepes.

Place the ricotta, cherries, yogurt, powdered sugar, and zest in a small bowl. Stir to combine.

Set out one crepe and top with 2 tablespoons of the filling. Roll and transfer to a plate. Repeat with the remaining crepes and filling. Serve immediately.

(2 FILLED CREPES) 430 CALORIES, 22 G PROTEIN, 14 G FAT (5 G SATURATED), 55 G CARBOHY-DRATES, 5 G FIBER, 319 MG SODIUM

BAKED EGGS WITH KALE AND PROSCIUTTO

SERVES 4 • SUPERFOODS: Eggs, Kale, Parmesan

Want to impress a guest (or simply wow yourself)? Crispy kale and savory prosciutto elevate an otherwise everyday bacon-and-egg breakfast to gourmet status. Clean your plate and you'll take in more than a full day's worth of vitamin C, which helps your body burn fat for fuel.

> Olive oil cooking spray
> 4 cups chopped kale
> 1/2 cup grated Parmesan
> 4 eggs
> 2 slices (1 ounce) prosciutto, excess fat removed
> 4 slices whole-grain bread, toasted
> 1/2 teaspoon freshly ground black pepper

Heat the oven to 400°F. On the stovetop, heat a large oven-safe skillet over high heat. Remove from the heat, coat with cooking spray, and return to the heat. Add the kale and cook 1 minute, turning often. Sprinkle the Parmesan over the kale and place the skillet in the oven.

Heat a second large oven-safe skillet over high heat. Remove from the heat, coat with cooking spray, and return to the heat. Crack the eggs gently into the skillet, sunny-side up, and cook for about 30 seconds, until the edges of the eggs start to cook. Carefully move the eggs aside and add the prosciutto to the skillet. Slide the skillet into the oven next to the kale-filled skillet.

Bake 3 to 4 minutes, until the kale and prosciutto are crispy and the white of the egg is cooked through. Remove both skillets from the oven. Place the toast on plates and top the four slices with 1/2 slice of prosciutto, 1 cup of kale, and 1 egg. Sprinkle with pepper and serve.

343 CALORIES, 17 G PROTEIN, 9 G FAT (4 G SATURATED), 25 G CARBOHYDRATES, 4 G FIBER, 710 MG SODIUM

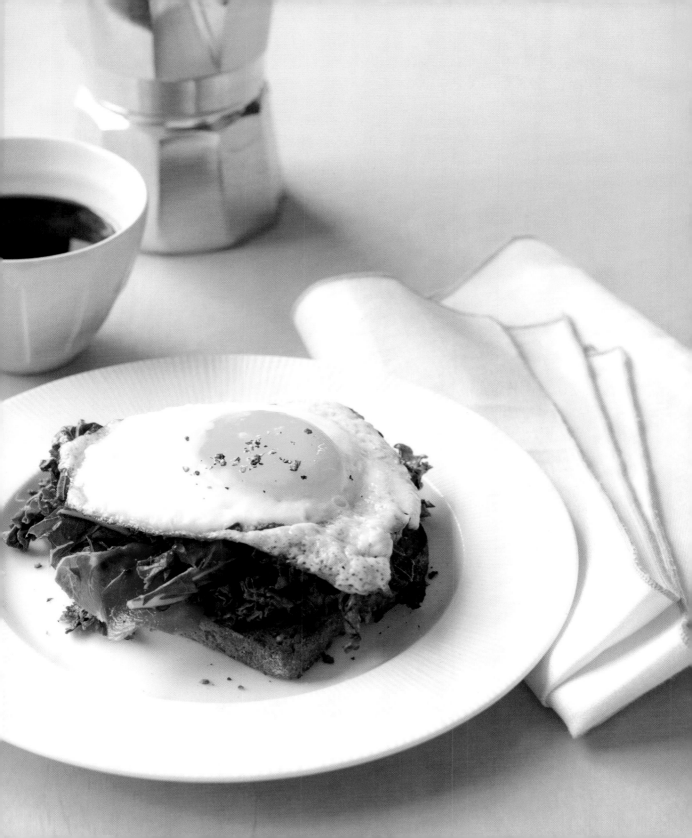

BLUEBERRY "ICE CREAM" SHAKE

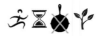

SERVES 1 • SUPERFOODS: Avocado, Blueberries, Yogurt

Ice cream for breakfast? That's what your taste buds will think! Avocado has an ice-cream–like, rich texture, except it offers slimming monounsaturated fat and fiber instead of unhealthy saturated fat. Don't worry, the taste of sweet, icy blueberries, vanilla, and tangy yogurt prevail.

> 1 cup frozen blueberries
> $^1/_2$ cup plain low-fat yogurt
> $^1/_2$ cup skim milk
> $^1/_4$ cup avocado (about $^1/_4$ Hass avocado)
> 4 ice cubes
> 1 tablespoon granulated sugar
> $^1/_2$ teaspoon vanilla extract

Place all ingredients in a blender and process until smooth. Serve immediately.

354 CALORIES, 18 G PROTEIN, 11 G FAT (2 G SATURATED), 50 G CARBOHYDRATES, 7 G FIBER, 107 MG SODIUM

GREEN TEA CHOCOLATE CHIP SMOOTHIE

SERVES 1 • SUPERFOODS: Dark Chocolate, Kiwifruit, Yogurt

Sipping the same standard smoothie every morning can get berry boring. Mix things up with sweet kiwifruit and mellow green tea without . . . oh, who are we fooling? It's all about the chocolate!

1 small banana
$\frac{1}{2}$ cup plain, low-fat yogurt
$\frac{1}{2}$ cup brewed green tea, chilled
1 small kiwi, peeled
2 ice cubes
2 tablespoons 70% cacao chocolate (break up a bar)
1 tablespoon granulated sugar

Place all ingredients in a blender and process until smooth. Serve immediately.

386 CALORIES, 10 G PROTEIN, 9 G FAT (5 G SATURATED), 74 G CARBOHYDRATES, 6 G FIBER, 92 MG SODIUM

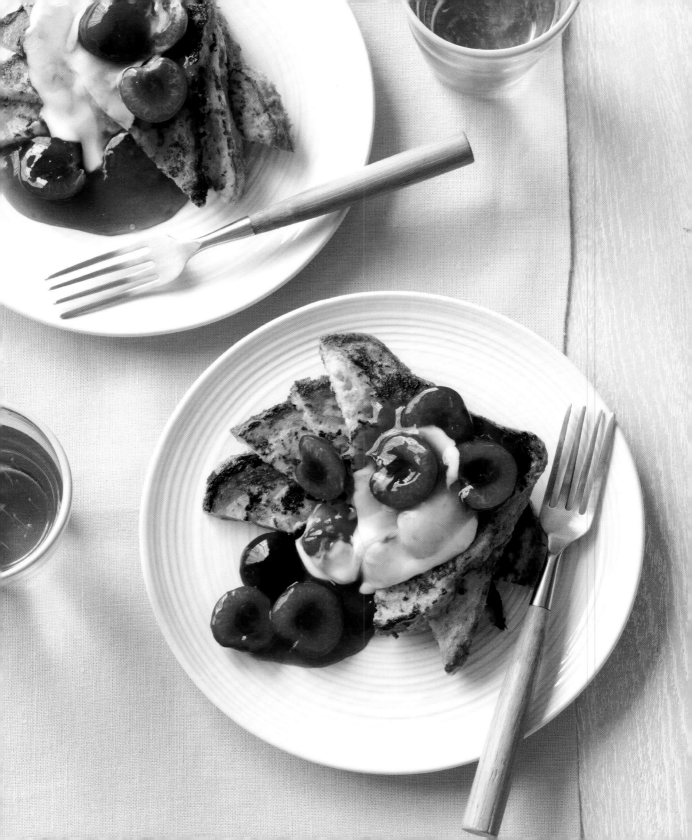

FRENCH TOAST WITH AMARETTO CHERRY SYRUP

SERVES 4 • SUPERFOODS: Cherries, Eggs, Yogurt

French toast is usually saturated with calories, but this version manages to cut out a big chunk while replacing them with more flavor, fiber, and protein disguised as finger-licking syrup and creamy topping. Your corner diner's got nothing on this!

¹⁄₄ cup plain, low-fat Greek yogurt

¹⁄₂ cup powdered sugar, divided

1 cup frozen or fresh cherries, chopped

1 cup water

2 tablespoons amaretto liqueur or ¹⁄₂ teaspoon almond extract

1 tablespoon cornstarch

3 eggs

1 ¹⁄₂ cups skim milk

1 teaspoon vanilla extract

8 slices whole-grain bread

Olive oil cooking spray

Place the yogurt and half of the powdered sugar in a small bowl. Stir together well and set aside.

Place the cherries, water, amaretto or extract, cornstarch, and remaining powdered sugar in a small saucepan. Simmer over low heat 5 to 6 minutes, stirring often, until a thick sauce forms. Remove from the heat and set aside.

Place the eggs, milk, and vanilla in a shallow bowl and whisk well. Dip each slice of bread in the mixture, pressing slightly with the back of a fork to allow the bread to soak up the egg mixture. Transfer to a plate.

Heat two large skillets over high heat. Remove each skillet from the heat, coat with cooking spray, and return to the heat. Reduce the heat to medium. Add four slices of the soaked bread to each skillet and cook 3 to 4 minutes, until the bread is golden. Flip and cook 2 to 3 minutes more, or until the second side is golden and the bread is firm in the center. Place two slices on each plate and top with a tablespoon of the sweetened yogurt and a quarter of the cherry mixture. Serve immediately.

(2 SLICES) 364 CALORIES, 17 G PROTEIN, 6 G FAT (1 G SATURATED), 61 G CARBOHYDRATES, 7 G FIBER, 438 MG SODIUM

PARMESAN BASIL FRITTATA

SERVES 4 • SUPERFOODS: Artichokes, Broccoli, Eggs, Olive Oil, Parmesan

Good thing this cheesy frittata reheats well; with portion sizes that defy diet logic, you may end up with leftovers. It maintains a low-calorie profile thanks to high-fiber, low-energy-dense superfoods that add bulk to your plate, not your weight.

6 eggs

4 sprigs basil, stem discarded, leaves chopped

1/2 cup finely grated Parmesan

2 tablespoons extra-virgin olive oil

2 cups broccoli florets, chopped

4 ounces frozen artichokes hearts, defrosted, chopped
 (about 1 cup)

1/2 cup chopped roasted red pepper

4 slices whole-grain bread, toasted

Heat the oven to 400°F. Place the eggs, basil, and Parmesan in a large bowl. Whisk to combine and set aside. Heat a medium-size, oven-safe skillet over medium heat. Add the olive oil and the broccoli and cook 2 to 3 minutes, stirring often, until the broccoli starts to soften.

> **TABLE FOR 1?**
>
> Eat your serving, then pack up the remaining three for quickie meals later in the week. Place on a bed of greens and add 1/2 cup guacamole for a filling lunch or dinner.

Add the egg mixture to the pan. Scatter the artichokes and red pepper over the eggs and slide the skillet into the oven. Bake 8 to 10 minutes, until the edges are firm to the touch. Remove the skillet from the oven and allow the frittata to cool 5 minutes in the pan. Loosen the inside edges with a metal spatula and flip the frittata out and onto a plate. Slice into four wedges and serve immediately with toast.

(1 SLICE FRITTATA PLUS 1 SLICE TOAST) 366 CALORIES, 19 G PROTEIN, 20 G FAT (6 G SATU-RATED), 29 G CARBOHYDRATES, 6 G FIBER, 665 MG SODIUM

PROTEIN-PACKED SMOOTHIE

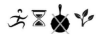

SERVES 1 • SUPERFOODS: Cherries, Edamame, Yogurt

Save powder for setting your makeup—yogurt and edamame give this thick, icy shake plenty of real-food protein power to help you build calorie-sizzling lean muscle and breeze right past the morning munchies. Plus, the cherries feed your sweet tooth, even as they fight fat with fiber and antioxidants.

1 cup plain, low-fat yogurt

1 cup frozen cherries

$1/3$ cup frozen shelled edamame, defrosted

$1/3$ cup skim milk

$1/4$ teaspoon almond extract

3 ice cubes

Place all ingredients in a blender and process until smooth. Serve immediately.

379 CALORIES, 22 G PROTEIN, 6 G FAT (3 G SATURATED), 60 G CARBOHYDRATES, 5 G FIBER, 211 MG SODIUM

CHEF'S NOTE:
Unlike fruit, which can go straight from the freezer to the blender, edamame must be thoroughly thawed first. Since they contain protein, they won't blend well while frozen.

STEAK AND EGGS RANCHEROS

SERVES 4 • SUPERFOODS: Eggs, Lentils, Steak

Holy protein, Batman! Lean flank steak, stick-to-your-ribs lentils, and satiating eggs add up to 30 grams of protein per serving, turning this spicy super breakfast into a metabolism blaster that—*POW!*—delivers a major blow to body fat.

8 ounces flank steak

1/4 teaspoon salt

Olive oil cooking spray

4 eggs

4 small whole-grain soft tortillas

1 cup cooked lentils

2 thin slices pepper jack cheese
    (about 1.5 ounces)

4 tablespoons salsa

a few sprigs of parsley (if desired)

> **TABLE FOR 1?**
>
> If you have leftover steak, use it with 1 egg, 1/4 cup lentils, and 1 tablespoon each shredded cheese and salsa.

Heat a skillet over high heat. Sprinkle the flank steak with the salt. Coat both sides of the flank steak with cooking spray and place it in the skillet. Reduce the heat to low and cook about 15 minutes, turning once or twice, until the steak is well browned and pink (not red) in the center. Transfer the steak to a cutting board to rest.

Heat a second skillet over high heat. Remove from the heat and coat with cooking spray. Return to the stove and carefully break the eggs into the pan, sunny-side up. Cook the eggs 3 minutes (do not flip).

Toast the tortillas in a toaster oven (or in an oven heated to 350°F). Transfer one tortilla to each of four plates. Top with 1/4 cup of the lentils, a quarter of the cheese, 1 tablespoon of the salsa, and 1 egg. Thinly slice the flank steak and add it to the plate. Garnish it with parsley, if desired, and serve.

352 CALORIES, 30 G PROTEIN, 12 G FAT (5 G SATURATED), 35 G CARBOHYDRATES, 12 G FIBER, 717 MG SODIUM

CHEF'S NOTE:
Spice is nice! Salsa weighs in at a slim 4 calories per tablespoon, so if you want to spoon on extra, go for it!

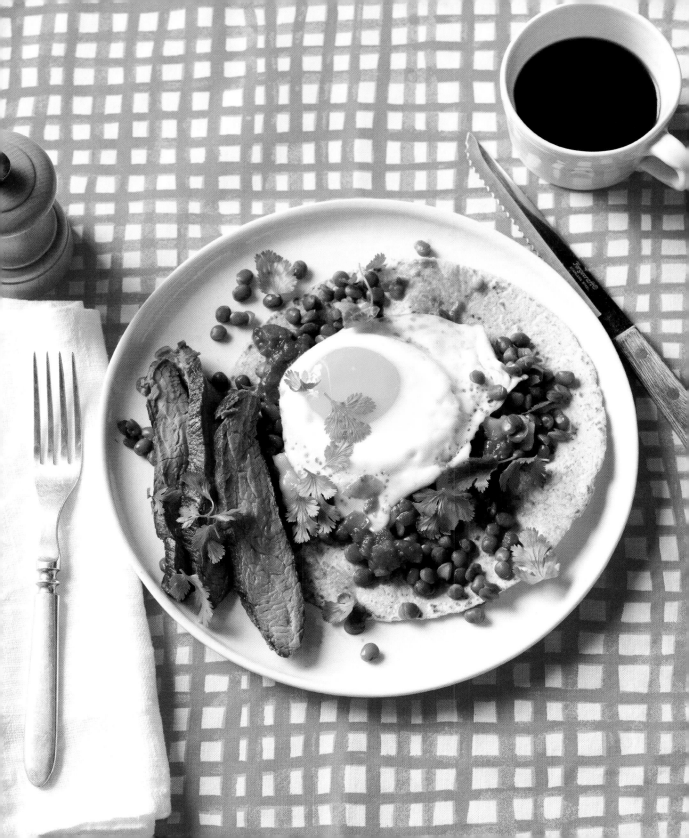

CHEESY BREAKFAST POCKET

Makes 8 Pockets • SUPERFOODS: Broccoli, Parmesan

The freezer-section versions of these one-handed meals can be so dinky, you could tuck them into *your* pocket! Here, gooey mozzarella and Parmesan burst from the soft, chewy homemade version, along with bite after bite of fresh broccoli, so you get a substantially bigger portion for less fat and loads more flab-torching vitamin C.

1 pound whole-wheat pizza dough, defrosted
1/2 cup whole-wheat pastry flour or soft whole-wheat
    flour (for rolling)
4 cups broccoli florets, chopped
16 ounces grated part-skim mozzarella (4 cups)
1/2 cup grated Parmesan
1/2 cup spicy or mild salsa

Heat the oven to 400°F. Cut the pizza dough into eight equal portions. Using 1 tablespoon of whole-wheat flour, roll each out into an 8 × 4-inch rectangle. In the center of each rectangle, place 1/2 cup broccoli, 1/2 cup mozzarella, 1 tablespoon Parmesan, and 1 tablespoon of salsa.

Fold the edges of each rectangle over to form a square and pinch to close. Bake 12 to 14 minutes, until the top is golden and the dough is firm to the touch. Remove from the oven and cool 5 minutes before serving. Cool completely before storing refrigerated in an airtight container up to 3 days.

 (1 POCKET) 317 CALORIES, 21 G PROTEIN, 12 G FAT (7 G SATURATED), 32 G CARBOHYDRATES, 2 G FIBER, 777 MG SODIUM

CHEF'S NOTE:
Despite a hefty portion size, calories are light—add 1/2 banana
to round up to about 366 calories, if desired.

APPLE ALMOND OAT MUFFINS

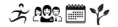

Makes 12 muffins • SUPERFOODS: Almond Butter, Apples, Eggs, Oats, Quinoa

Watch out, country belles, these beauties look as pretty and are as sweet and moist as classic, blue-ribbon baked goods. The ultimate prize, however, is the lean, healthy figure you'll achieve by eating them.

Olive oil cooking spray
$3/4$ cup whole-wheat pastry flour
    or soft whole-wheat flour
$3/4$ cup oat flour
1 teaspoon baking soda
$1/2$ teaspoon baking powder
$1/2$ teaspoon ground cinnamon
$1/4$ teaspoon salt
$1/2$ cup brown sugar
$1/4$ cup almond butter
1 egg
1 cup cooked quinoa
1 cup grated apple, peel
    included
$1/2$ cup skim milk
1 teaspoon almond extract

Heat the oven to 350°F. Coat a twelve-cup muffin tin with cooking spray, or line with paper liners. Combine the flours, baking soda, baking powder, cinnamon, and salt in a large bowl. Stir well and set aside.

Place the brown sugar and almond butter in a large bowl. Using a wooden spoon, mix until smooth. Stir in the egg. Add the quinoa, apple, milk, and almond extract and mix well. Add the flour mixture and stir until just combined. Do not overmix.

Fill each muffin cup three-fourths full. Bake for 20 to 25 minutes, or until the muffins spring back to the touch when pressed. Transfer to a wire rack to cool. Store in an airtight container for up to 3 days.

TABLE FOR 1?

Halve the recipe and fill only three cups each in two muffin tins. Bake one pan now (store extras up to 3 days in an airtight container); cover the other in foil and stash it in the freezer for up to 2 weeks. When you're ready to bake, transfer the tin directly into your heated oven and bake 22 to 27 minutes.

(1 MUFFIN) 153 CALORIES, 4 G PROTEIN, 5 G FAT (0 G SATURATED), 25 G CARBOHYDRATES, 2 G FIBER, 305 MG SODIUM

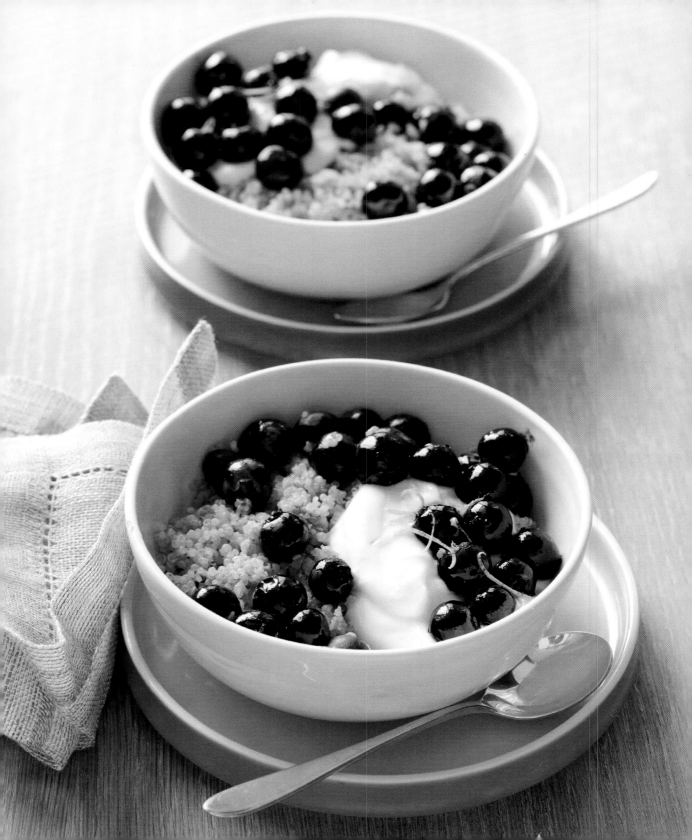

BLUEBERRIES AND CREAM QUINOA

SERVES 1 • SUPERFOODS: Almond Butter, Blueberries, Quinoa, Yogurt

Boxed cereal can't compete with the fat-melting, stomach-filling nutrients that go into this hearty bowl—protein, fiber, calcium, healthy fats, and antioxidants—nor its rich mix of sweet and zingy flavors.

$^1/_2$ cup cooked quinoa, warm or at room temperature

2 teaspoons almond butter

$^1/_2$ cup plain, low-fat Greek yogurt

1 tablespoon powdered sugar

$^1/_2$ teaspoon vanilla extract

1 cup fresh or frozen blueberries, thawed

1 teaspoon lemon zest

Place the quinoa in a cereal bowl. Add the almond butter and mix well. Set aside.

In a separate bowl, mix together the yogurt, powdered sugar, and vanilla extract; spoon over the quinoa mixture. Top with blueberries and lemon zest and serve.

340 CALORIES, 16 G PROTEIN, 10 G FAT (2 G SATURATED), 49 G CARBOHYDRATES, 6 G FIBER, 87 MG SODIUM

CHEF'S NOTE:

If you have a batch of quinoa on hand, you can put breakfast on the table in minutes. You can also mix this up the night before, cover, and let chill in the fridge for a speedy morning meal.

EGG PUFFS THREE WAYS

A basic, quick-baking batter is a blank canvas for flavor—and fat fighting, especially when it's this low in calories! You can add more servings to increase your calories—and don't be afraid to experiment by adding in other veggies and lean protein.

Basic Egg Puffs

SERVES 4 (makes 8 puffs) • SUPERFOODS: Eggs, Oats, Parmesan

Olive oil cooking spray
$1/4$ cup oat flour
$1/2$ teaspoon baking soda
8 eggs
$1/2$ cup grated Parmesan

Heat the oven to 400°F. Coat a twelve-cup muffin tin with cooking spray. Place the flour and baking soda in a large bowl and stir well to combine. Add the eggs and the Parmesan and whisk well to combine. Pour into the muffin tin, filling each of eight cups three-fourths full. Bake 5 to 7 minutes, until the tops begin to brown and the egg puffs up. Remove from the oven, run a knife along the inside edge to loosen each puff, and transfer to a plate. Serve immediately.

 (2 PUFFS) 208 CALORIES, 17 G PROTEIN, 12 G FAT (4 G SATURATED), 5 G CARBOHYDRATES, 0.5 G FIBER, 452 MG SODIUM

Cheese and Broccoli Puffs

SERVES 6 (makes 12 puffs) • SUPERFOODS: Broccoli, Eggs, Oats, Parmesan

Olive oil cooking spray
$1/4$ cup oat flour
$1/2$ teaspoon baking soda
8 eggs
1 cup broccoli florets, chopped
$1/2$ cup grated Parmesan
$1/3$ cup grated part-skim mozzarella

Heat the oven to 400°F. Coat a twelve-cup muffin tin with cooking spray. Place the flour and baking soda in a large bowl and stir well to combine. Add the eggs, broccoli, Parmesan, and mozzarella. Pour into the muffin tin, filling each of the twelve cups three-fourths full. Bake 12 to 14 minutes, until the tops begin to brown and the egg puffs up. Remove from the oven, run a knife along the inside edge to loosen each puff, and transfer to a plate. Serve immediately.

 (2 PUFFS) 216 CALORIES, 17 G PROTEIN, 12 G FAT (4 G SATURATED), 5 G CARBOHYDRATES, 0.5 G FIBER, 452 MG SODIUM

Smoked Wild Salmon and Broccoli Puffs

SERVES 6 (makes 12 puffs) • SUPERFOODS: Broccoli, Eggs, Parmesan, Wild Salmon

Olive oil cooking spray
1/4 cup oat flour
1/2 teaspoon baking soda
8 eggs
1 cup broccoli florets, chopped
1/2 cup grated Parmesan
2 ounces smoked wild salmon, chopped

Heat the oven to 400°F. Coat a sixteen-cup muffin tin with cooking spray. Place the flour and baking soda in a large bowl and stir well to combine. Add the eggs, broccoli, Parmesan, and smoked salmon. Pour into the muffin tin, filling each of the cups three-fourths full. Bake 12 to 14 minutes, until the tops begin to brown and the egg puffs up. Remove from the oven, run a knife along the inside edge to loosen each puff, and transfer to a plate. Serve immediately.

 (2 PUFFS) 155 CALORIES, 14 G PROTEIN, 9 G FAT (3 G SATURATED), 4 G CARBOHYDRATES, 1 G FIBER, 496 MG SODIUM

CHEF'S NOTE:
The puffs containing broccoli yield more because the veggie adds more volume. Whichever type of puff you choose, feel free to add a piece of fresh fruit to bump up your meal's fiber and calorie count.

DEVIL'S FOOD CHERRY CHOCOLATE BREAKFAST MUFFINS

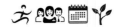

Makes 12 muffins • SUPERFOODS: Cherries, Coffee, Dark Chocolate, Eggs, Oats, Olive Oil, Yogurt

Most muffins have so much fat and sugar, they are really dessert in disguise. The opposite is true here: With fiber-rich whole grains standing in for insulin-spiking refined white flour, plus yogurt and olive oil subbing for butter, this surprisingly fudgy cake tastes almost too decadent to eat first thing. Almost.

$^1/_2$ cup boiling water

6 tablespoons unsweetened natural cocoa powder

2 teaspoons finely ground coffee

1 teaspoon vanilla extract

1 $^1/_4$ cups oat flour

$^3/_4$ cup whole-wheat pastry flour

1 $^1/_2$ teaspoons baking soda

$^1/_4$ teaspoon salt

$^3/_4$ cup granulated sugar

$^1/_4$ cup light olive oil

1 egg

$^1/_2$ cup plain reduced-fat Greek yogurt

2 cups fresh cherries (or frozen, thawed), chopped

Heat the oven to 400°F. Line a twelve-cup muffin tin with muffin papers. Place the water in a small bowl and add the cocoa powder, coffee, and vanilla extract. Whisk well, until a thick mixture forms. Set aside to cool for 5 minutes.

In a large bowl, mix together the flours, baking soda, and salt.

In a separate large bowl, add the sugar, olive oil, and egg. Whisk to combine well. Add the yogurt and stir with a wooden spoon until just combined. Add half the flour

> ### SWEET SURPRISE!
>
> Indulging in chocolate or other treats in the morning may actually help you control cravings and lose more weight than if you saved dessert for after dinner or skipped it altogether, say researchers at Tel Aviv University. Dieters who punctuated healthy, balanced, protein-rich breakfasts with cake, chocolate, or cookies shed about 40 more pounds over thirty-two weeks than those who didn't enjoy a morning treat.

mixture and stir until just combined. Add the chocolate mixture and stir a few times. Add the remaining flour mixture and cherries, stir until combined. Do not overmix.

Spoon the batter into the muffin tin, filling each cup almost to the top. Bake 10 to 15 minutes, until the muffins spring back to the touch. Remove the muffins from the tin and cool completely on a wire rack.

 (1 MUFFIN) 182 CALORIES, 4 G PROTEIN, 7 G FAT (1 G SATURATED), 29 G CARBOHYDRATES, 3 G FIBER, 215 MG SODIUM

CHEF'S NOTE:
If you want to transform these muffins into a true dessert, add ½ cup semisweet chocolate chips to the batter. The damage? About 30 waist-friendly calories each.

CINNAMON SWEET POTATO MUFFINS

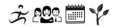

Makes 12 muffins • SUPERFOODS: Eggs, Oats, Olive Oil,
Pumpkin Seeds, Sweet Potatoes

Hiding veggies in baked goods gives flab the slip by driving down calories and fat while boosting your intake of essential waist-trimming vitamins. What isn't sneaking around at all: the irresistible moistness and flavor of the warm, finished product.

1 cup packed brown sugar, divided
1/2 cup pumpkin seeds
2 teaspoons ground cinnamon, divided
1/4 cup olive oil
1 egg
2 teaspoons vanilla extract

3 cups peeled, grated sweet potato (about 10 ounces)
1 cup whole-wheat pastry flour
1 cup oat flour
2 teaspoons baking powder
1/4 teaspoon salt
1/2 cup skim milk, divided

Heat the oven to 350°F. Line a twelve-cup muffin tin with muffin papers. In a small bowl, place half the brown sugar, the pumpkin seeds, and half the cinnamon; mix well. Set aside to use for the topping.

In a large bowl, place the remaining brown sugar and cinnamon, olive oil, egg, and vanilla extract. Mix with a wooden spoon. Add the sweet potato and mix well. Set aside.

In a separate large bowl, place the flours, baking powder, and salt and mix well. Add half of the flour mixture to the wet brown sugar mixture. Stir until just combined. Add half the milk and stir again, but do not overmix. Repeat.

Fill each muffin cup three-fourths full. Press 2 teaspoons of the dry brown sugar and pumpkin seed topping onto the surface of each muffin. Bake for 20 to 25 minutes, or until the muffins spring back when pressed. Remove the muffins from the tin and transfer to a wire rack until cool. Store in an airtight container for up to 3 days.

(1 MUFFIN) 215 CALORIES, 5 G PROTEIN, 9 G FAT (1 G SATURATED), 31 G CARBOHYDRATES, 3 G FIBER, 80 MG SODIUM

CHEF'S NOTE:
A stand-up box grater makes quick work of the spuds, but using a food processor with the grater attachment speeds your prep even more.

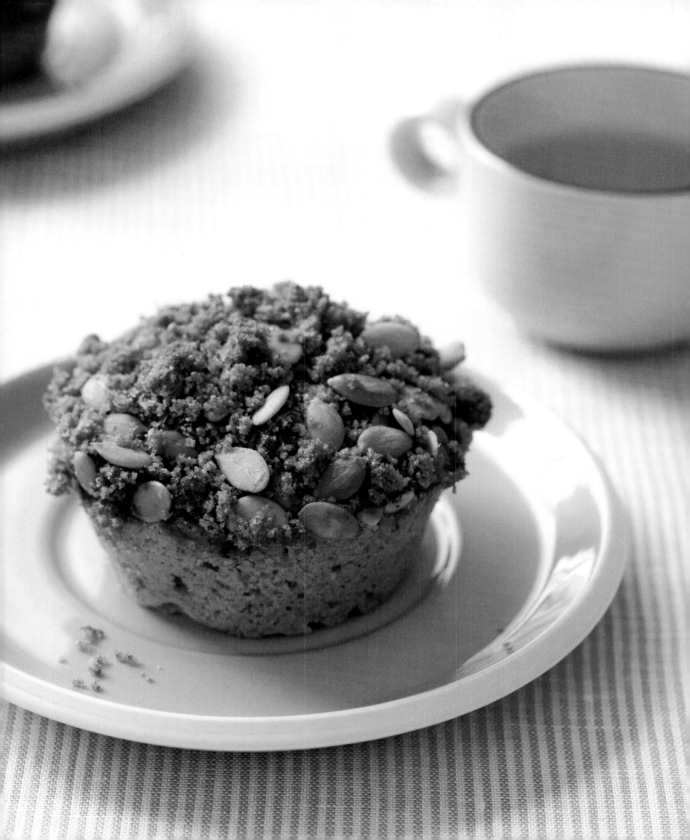

SUPER-MOIST BREAKFAST BANANA BREAD

SERVES 12 • SUPERFOODS: Eggs, Oats, Quinoa, Yogurt

Sweet, ripe bananas may get all the glory in this remake of the classic, but quinoa is the unsung star of the show. The whole grain prevents the cakey bread from drying out and adds extra protein, fiber, and nutrients like manganese, which helps keep your bones strong.

Nonstick cooking spray

1 cup oat flour

1/2 cup whole-wheat pastry flour or
   soft white whole-wheat flour

3 tablespoons ground flax

2 teaspoons baking powder

1/4 teaspoon baking soda

1/8 teaspoon salt

3/4 cup granulated sugar

5 tablespoons unsalted butter,
   room temperature

2 eggs

1 1/2 cups mashed banana (about
   4 small bananas)

1/2 cup cooked quinoa

1/2 cup plain low-fat Greek yogurt

Heat the oven 350°F. Line a 2-pound loaf pan with aluminum foil. Coat with cooking spray.

Place the flours, flax, baking powder, baking soda, and salt in a large bowl, and whisk to combine. Set aside.

In a separate large bowl, place the sugar and butter. With an electric mixer on high speed, beat the sugar and butter until the mixture is light yellow and fluffy. Reduce the speed to medium and add the eggs one at a time, until combined.

Reduce the speed to low and add the banana, quinoa, and yogurt; mix until just combined. Set the mixer aside. Add the flour mixture. Using a wooden spoon, stir until just combined. Spoon the batter into the prepared loaf pan and bake 50 to 55 minutes, until the center of the bread springs back to the touch. If the bread browns too quickly, cover the top loosely with aluminum foil.

Transfer to a wire rack and cool 5 minutes in the pan. Lift the bread out of the pan and cool completely on a wire rack before slicing. Wrap tightly in aluminum foil and store refrigerated for up to 5 days.

(1 SLICE) 193 CALORIES, 4 G PROTEIN, 8 G FAT (4 G SATURATED), 29 G CARBOHYDRATES, 2 G FIBER, 88 MG SODIUM

CHEF'S NOTE:
Got overly ripe, brown bananas? Stick them in the freezer for up to a week, until you're ready to make this recipe. Defrost in the fridge before using.

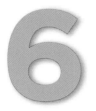

AMAZINGLY SLIM AND SATISFYING MAIN MEALS

PICTURE THIS: YOU DECIDE YOU'RE GOING TO READ MORE, BUT choose a tome that makes *War and Peace* seem like a fun page-turner. You'd never do that, of course, because you'd be setting yourself up to fail. That's what happens when you decide to lose weight by eating typical diet foods or following a quickie fix like a cleanse. Plain steamed veggies, lemon juice and cayenne mixes—sure, the pounds will come off quickly, but they'll fly back on once you give up the regimen. And you *will* give up, because restrictive plans suck the joy out of eating and sap your motivation.

Now imagine yourself digging into Spicy Steak Tacos, Prosciutto-Wrapped Chicken with Gingered Apple Goji Chutney, or Mushroom-Turkey Meatballs with Angel-Hair Pasta. Think of the Drop 10 recipes as the *50 Shades of Grey* of diet food—irresistible, surprising, sometimes spicy, and easy to get through. Yep, aside from looking and tasting unpredictably delicious, each dish in this chapter is super simple and quick to make. Look for the ⧗ for recipes you can prep quickly or ▮ for those that freeze and reheat well.

These main events have a few other things going for them, too. Research from the University of Texas shows that people tend to eat 150 percent more in the evening. These recipes give you the big portions you want, but for only about 450 calories. By spreading out your calories evenly throughout the day, you'll be able to keep nighttime cravings at bay. Too bad reading important books like *War and Peace* isn't this easy.

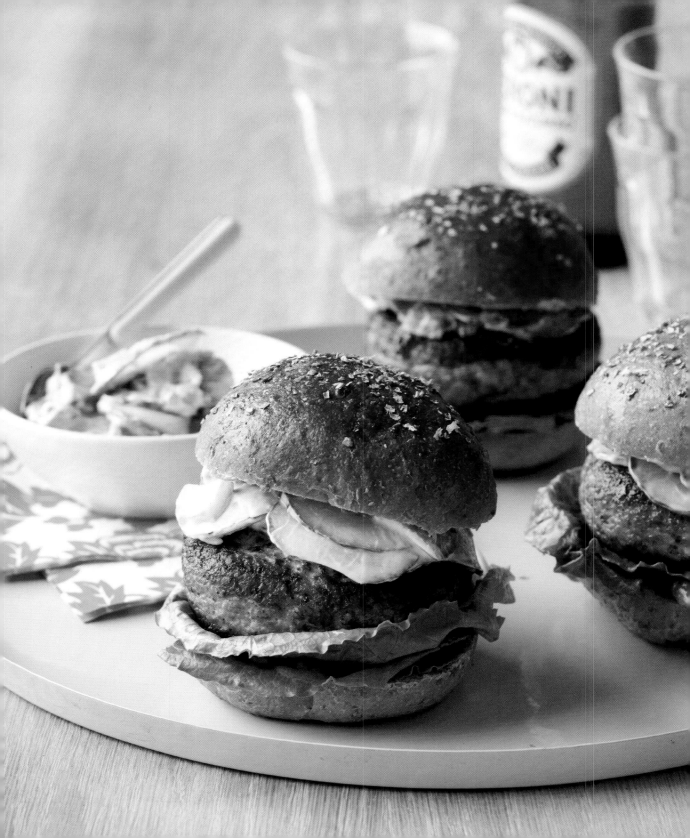

SPICY CHICKEN BURGER WITH COOL AVOCADO-CUCUMBER TOPPING

SERVES 4 • SUPERFOODS: Avocado, Edamame, Mushrooms, Olive Oil, Yogurt

In typical diet meals, flavor and portion size tend to be the collateral damage of calorie trimming. But meaty, mighty mushrooms—a mere 20 calories per sliced cup—rescue all in this burger, locking in juicy moisture while beefing up your serving size.

¼ cup plain, low-fat Greek yogurt

1 teaspoon white wine vinegar

½ teaspoon granulated sugar

½ small red onion, cut in half

1 ripe avocado, cut into 1-inch chunks

1 cup thinly sliced cucumber

1 portobello mushroom cap, gills removed, quartered

1 cup frozen shelled edamame, defrosted

2 garlic cloves, peeled and quartered

2 6-ounce boneless, skinless chicken breasts, quartered

2 tablespoons reduced-sodium soy sauce

¼–½ teaspoon cayenne pepper

1 tablespoon olive oil

4 whole-wheat English muffins or buns, split and toasted

lettuce (if desired)

Heat the oven to 400°F. In a small bowl, place the yogurt, vinegar, and sugar; whisk well. Dice half the red onion into ½-inch pieces. Add it to the yogurt mixture; add the avocado and cucumber and toss to coat.

Place the mushrooms, edamame, garlic, and remaining onion in a food processor. Process until finely chopped. Add the chicken, soy sauce, and cayenne. Pulse about twelve times to chop the chicken and blend the mushrooms and edamame into the meat. Form into four equal patties.

Heat a large skillet over high heat. Add the olive oil and the burger patties and cook 4 to 5 minutes, turning once, until both sides are browned. Slide the skillet with the burger into the oven. Bake 12 to 14 minutes, until the burgers are cooked through. Place lettuce, if desired, on English muffins, and top with a burger and the avocado mixture.

THE DISH

436 CALORIES, 31 G PROTEIN, 20 G FAT (4 G SATURATED), 36 G CARBOHYDRATES, 7 G FIBER, 597 MG SODIUM

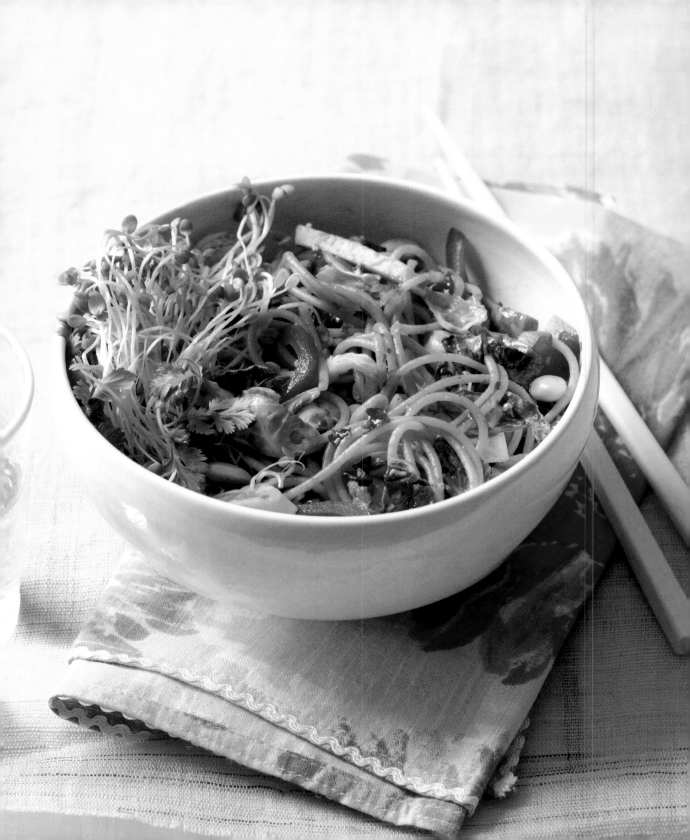

VEGGIE PAD THAI

SERVES 4 • SUPERFOODS: Edamame, Eggs, Olive Oil, Peanuts,
Whole-Grain Pasta

Tangy lime, spicy chili, rich peanuts—the Drop 10 version of this take-out favorite packs all the flavors you crave, plus so much more: 178 percent of your daily vitamin C (a fat burner!), 34 percent of your daily iron, plus a substantial helping of fiber.

Olive oil cooking spray

2 eggs, beaten

4 garlic cloves, minced

3 tablespoons brown sugar

2 limes, zested and juiced

1 tablespoon light olive oil, divided

1 tablespoon hot sauce, such as sambal

4 teaspoons fish sauce

8 ounces dry, whole-wheat spaghetti, cooked according to the package instructions

1 pint brussels sprouts, roughly chopped

1 red bell pepper, cored and thinly sliced

1 cup frozen, shelled edamame

2 cups broccoli sprouts

½ cup packed cilantro leaves

¼ cup dry-roasted, unsalted peanuts, chopped

Heat a medium skillet over medium-high heat. Remove from the heat, coat with cooking spray, and return to the stove. Add the eggs to the pan and cook 30 to 40 seconds, until the edges brown. Flip the eggs with a metal spatula and cook 1 minute, until cooked through. Transfer to a cutting board.

In a large bowl, add the garlic, brown sugar, lime zest and juice, half the olive oil, hot sauce, and fish sauce. Whisk well. Add the cooked pasta to the bowl and set aside.

Add the remaining olive oil to the skillet over medium heat. Add the brussels sprouts and bell pepper. Cook 3 to 4 minutes, stirring often, until the pepper softens. Add the edamame and cook 1 minute, until they defrost. Add the vegetables to the pasta mixture. Thinly slice the egg and add it to the bowl. Toss well and divide among four dishes. Top each with ½ cup of broccoli sprouts, 2 tablespoons of cilantro, and a sprinkle of peanuts. Serve immediately.

THE DISH

477 CALORIES, 24 G PROTEIN, 14 G FAT (2 G SATURATED), 74 G CARBOHYDRATES, 10 G FIBER, 725 MG SODIUM

SPICY STEAK TACOS

SERVES 4 • SUPERFOODS: Goji Berries, Steak

Say *bienvenidos* to smaller jeans with this crispy, nutrient-rich feast. Fill up on three crunchy shells loaded with lean steak and fresh veggies for fewer calories than found in two fast-food tacos.

1 tomato, seeded and chopped

¼ cup goji berries

¼ red onion, minced (about 2 tablespoons)

¼ cup packed cilantro leaves, chopped

1 ounce chipotle chile en adobo, chopped (1 tablespoon
      chile with sauce)

1 lime, zested and juiced

1 teaspoon granulated sugar

¼ teaspoon salt

6 ounces pre-cooked flank steak, sliced into 12 thin strips

12 taco shells

2 slices (2 ounces) part-skim mozzarella, cut into thin
      strips

1 cup mesclun greens, chopped

Heat the oven to 300°F. To make the salsa, place the tomato, goji berries, red onion, cilantro, chipotle, lime zest and juice, sugar, and salt in a bowl. Stir well and set aside.

   Distribute the meat inside the shells. Add mozzarella to each. Warm the taco shells in the oven 8 to 10 minutes, until the cheese melts. Top each with salsa and serve.

THE DISH (3 FILLED TACOS) 344 CALORIES, 18 G PROTEIN, 15 G FAT (6 G SATURATED), 35 G CARBOHY-DRATES, 4 G FIBER, 464 MG SODIUM

GOJI LENTIL SALAD WITH CARAMELIZED ONIONS AND PINEAPPLE

SERVES 4 • SUPERFOODS: Edamame, Goji Berries, Lentils, Olive Oil

Food that looks as good as it tastes is doubly satisfying. The lentils and edamame in this fresh, colorful salad add fiber and protein to further tame hunger and cravings. No wonder one-note macaroni and potato salads are sides, while this one stars as a meal.

1 cup balsamic vinegar

2 tablespoons olive oil

1 onion, cut into rings

1 tablespoon brown sugar

$1/2$ teaspoon salt

1 cup dry lentils, cooked according to the package instructions

$1/4$ cup goji berries

1 cup pineapple cubes, finely chopped

1 cup frozen shelled edamame, defrosted

1 6-inch whole-wheat pita, cut into 8 wedges

Place the balsamic vinegar in a small saucepan and cook over medium heat about 5 minutes, until the liquid reduces by half and a dark liquid forms (the mixture will thicken as it cools). Set aside.

> **FEELING SAUCY?**
>
> Make a double batch of the balsamic reduction to keep on hand to drizzle on sautéed broccoli, kale, or mushrooms.

Heat a large skillet over medium-high heat. Add the olive oil, onion, brown sugar, and salt. Reduce the heat to low and cook 20 to 25 minutes, stirring often, until the onion softens and turns a golden brown. (If the onion sticks, add a few tablespoons of water to the pan.)

Place the cooked lentils in a large bowl. Add the gojis, pineapple, edamame, and caramelized onion. Toss to combine. Transfer to four plates and drizzle with the balsamic reduction. Serve immediately with pita.

THE DISH 443 CALORIES, 21 G PROTEIN, 10 G FAT (1 G SATURATED), 71 G CARBOHYDRATES, 20 G FIBER, 478 MG SODIUM

CHEF'S NOTE:
You can caramelize the onions and cook the lentils a day ahead.
Store in the fridge, then toss this salad together in minutes.

TRUFFLED MAC 'N' CHEESE

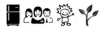

SERVES 4 • SUPERFOODS: Artichokes, Broccoli, Mushrooms, Olive Oil, Parmesan, Whole-Grain Pasta

Boxed mixes may be slightly faster to prep, but they can't compete in taste and fat fighting. This recipe packs a trio of creamy cheeses, fat-whittling fiber, and hunger-beating protein into every bite.

2 ounces (2 cups) dried mushrooms, any type

1 cup boiling water

2 tablespoons truffle oil or olive oil

3 tablespoons whole-wheat pastry flour

1/2 teaspoon salt

1/4 teaspoon freshly ground black pepper

1 cup skim milk

4 ounces shiitake mushrooms, stems discarded, caps thinly sliced

1 cup grated Fontina cheese (about 2 ounces; grate on a microplane)

1/2 cup grated Parmesan

1 ounce goat cheese

1 9-ounce package frozen artichoke hearts, defrosted and roughly chopped

6 ounces dry, whole-wheat macaroni, cooked according to the package instructions

1 head broccoli, cut into florets, stalk discarded, steamed

Rinse the dried mushrooms well under cold running water to remove dirt. Place in a small bowl along with 1 cup of boiling water. Allow to rest for 15 minutes, then drain, reserving 1/2 cup of the liquid.

Heat a large stockpot over medium heat. Add the truffle oil or olive oil, flour, salt, and black pepper. Cook 1 to 2 minutes, stirring often, until a thick paste forms. Reduce the heat to low, add half of the milk, and whisk well to create a soft paste. Whisk in the remaining milk and reserved mushroom liquid. Add the shiitakes and cook 2 to 3 minutes, stirring occasionally, until the mushrooms are soft and a thick mixture forms.

Add the Fontina, Parmesan, and goat cheese. Stir together well and cook 1 minute, until the cheese melts. Add the artichokes and cooked pasta. Stir well to coat. Serve immediately with the broccoli on the side.

THE DISH

(INCLUDES BROCCOLI) 469 CALORIES, 24 G PROTEIN, 17 G FAT (7 G SATURATED), 63 G CARBOHYDRATES, 11 G FIBER, 677 MG SODIUM

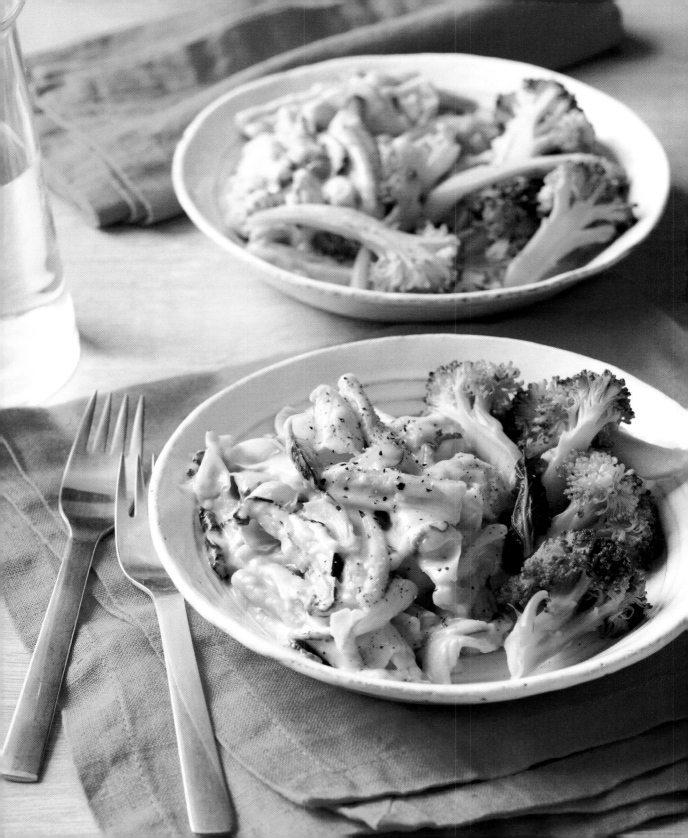

ALMOND BUTTER CHICKEN SATAY

SERVES 4 • SUPERFOODS: Almond Butter, Mushrooms, Yogurt

The creamy superfood dipping sauce, plus soba noodles and veggies, upgrades an otherwise ordinary appetizer to a lean, protein-powered meal.

24 small wooden skewers

2 skinless, boneless chicken breasts (12 ounces), cut into 12 thin strips

1 red bell pepper, cut into 2-inch cubes

1 5-ounce container mushrooms, stems removed

½ red onion, cut into 2-inch cubes

4 teaspoons curry powder, such as Madras

Olive oil cooking spray

4 ounces dry soba noodles, cooked according to the package instructions

SATAY SAUCE:

¼ cup almond butter

¼ cup coconut milk

¼ cup plain, low-fat Greek yogurt

1 lime, zested and juiced

1 tablespoon chili sauce, such as sambal or Sriracha

2 garlic cloves, minced

2 teaspoons fish sauce

½ teaspoon granulated sugar

Soak the skewers in water about 1 hour. Thread the chicken onto twelve of the skewers and set aside. Thread the red pepper, mushrooms, and red onion on the remaining skewers.

Heat a grill or grill pan over medium heat. Sprinkle the curry powder over the chicken and vegetable skewers. Coat them all with cooking spray. Place them on the grill and cook for 8 to 10 minutes, turning often, until the chicken is cooked through and the vegetables are tender.

PREPARE THE SATAY SAUCE:

Whisk together all ingredients. Serve as a dipping sauce, with the noodles on the side.

 THE DISH (6 SKEWERS, PLUS NOODLES) 387 CALORIES, 30 G PROTEIN, 16 G FAT (4 G SATURATED), 34 G CARBOHYDRATES, 6 G FIBER, 752 MG SODIUM

TUSCAN FENNEL WHITE BEAN SALAD

SERVES 4 • SUPERFOODS: Olive Oil, Parmesan, Sardines, Yogurt

Don't know beans? Don't miss out! Flush with slimming fiber and protein, energizing iron, and more, these legumes pair perfectly with the fat-sizzling superfoods in this no-cook dish.

$\frac{1}{2}$ cup grated Parmesan

2 lemons, zested and juiced

3 tablespoons extra-virgin olive oil

2 tablespoons plain low-fat yogurt

1 teaspoon hot sauce

1 teaspoon garlic powder

$\frac{1}{4}$ teaspoon freshly ground black pepper

$\frac{1}{4}$ teaspoon salt

6 cups baby arugula

1 large fennel bulb, shredded or thinly sliced

1 15-ounce can white beans, such as cannellini or navy, drained and rinsed well under cold running water

$\frac{1}{2}$ cup black olives, pitted, halved (16 pieces, or 8 pieces if using jumbo olives, such as Cerignola)

1 5-ounce can light tuna in springwater, drained

1 canned sardines in water, drained, chopped

4 ounces whole-wheat baguette, cut into 4 even hunks

BLOAT-BEATER

Rinsing canned beans washes away up to 40 percent of the sodium.

Place the Parmesan, lemon zest and juice, olive oil, yogurt, hot sauce, garlic powder, black pepper, and salt in a blender or mini chopper. Blend until smooth and set aside.

In a large bowl, toss the arugula, fennel, beans, olives, tuna, and sardines.

Divide the salad among four plates and drizzle each with the dressing. Serve immediately with the bread.

THE DISH (INCLUDING BREAD) 469 CALORIES, 29 G PROTEIN, 17 G FAT (4 G SATURATED), 56 G CARBOHYDRATES, 13 G FIBER, 799 MG SODIUM

CHEF'S NOTE:
Use a Japanese mandoline on the fennel to shorten prep time and produce elegantly slim slices.

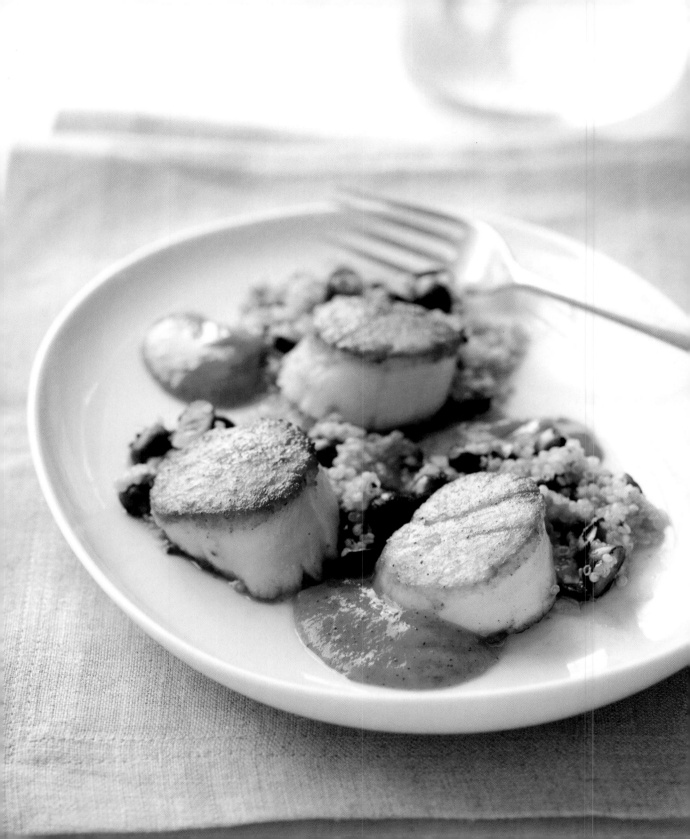

SCALLOP QUINOA WITH KIWI CILANTRO SAUCE

SERVES 4 • SUPERFOODS: Avocado, Blueberries, Kiwifruit, Oats, Olive Oil, Quinoa

Why save the fat-melting powers of super fruits for breakfast or snacks? Blueberries and kiwi team up with jalapeño to create slimming sweet-and-spicy flavors for this elegant, easy dish.

2 kiwis, peeled

$1/2$ avocado

$1/2$ small jalapeño, seeded and quartered

$1/4$ cup packed cilantro leaves, chopped

1 small lime, juiced (about $1/4$ cup juice)

$1 1/4$ cups dry quinoa, rinsed well under cold running water

1 cup blueberries, chopped

1 cup jarred salsa verde

$1/4$ cup oat flour

$1/2$ teaspoon paprika

1 pound large sea scallops (12–16 scallops)

2 tablespoons olive oil

Place the kiwis, avocado, jalapeño, cilantro, and lime juice in a blender and process until smooth. Set aside.

In a large serving bowl, gently toss together the quinoa, blueberries, and salsa verde.

Place the oat flour and paprika on a small plate, and mix with your clean fingertips. Press both sides of the scallops into the flour mixture.

Heat a large skillet over high heat. Add the olive oil. Add the flour-coated scallops and cook 2 minutes without moving. Once the scallops are golden on the underside, carefully turn them over and cook 1 minute. Transfer to the quinoa mixture and drizzle with the kiwi sauce. Serve immediately.

> ### SPEEDY GOURMET
> If you have precooked quinoa on hand, you can put this wow-worthy meal on the table in 15 minutes flat.

THE DISH 477 CALORIES, 23 G PROTEIN, 14 G FAT (2 G SATURATED), 58 G CARBOHYDRATES, 7 G FIBER, 755 MG SODIUM

SWEET POTATO PARMESAN SOUFFLÉ WITH ARUGULA SALAD

SERVES 4 • SUPERFOODS: Eggs, Goji Berries, Oats, Olive Oil, Parmesan, Sweet Potatoes

You say potato, we say potat-*no* to bland, boring diet food. These warm, fluffy, and cheesy spuds are balanced by crisp greens and chewy, tart gojis for a satisfying mix of textures and tastes. You'll hit more than one-third of your calcium needs while you eat, setting up your body for optimal fat burning.

3 large sweet potatoes, cut in half
1/2 cup grated Parmesan
1/2 cup skim milk
3 tablespoons oat flour

6 eggs
2 teaspoons baking soda
1/4 teaspoon salt

ARUGULA SALAD:
1 lemon, zested and juiced
2 tablespoons olive oil
6 cups baby arugula
1/4 cup goji berries

Heat the oven to 400°F. Poke the potatoes two or three times with a fork and place them on a baking sheet. Bake 45 to 50 minutes, until they are easily pierced with a knife, or are soft to the touch. Cool on the countertop for 5 minutes, then spoon the flesh into a large mixing bowl.

Add the Parmesan, milk, flour, eggs, baking soda, and salt. Using an electric mixer, beat on high speed 20 to 30 seconds, until smooth. Transfer the mixture to a 2-quart baking dish. Bake 24 to 30 minutes, until the soufflé puffs. Cool 5 minutes before cutting into and serving. Divide the soufflé among four plates.

PREPARE THE SALAD:
Place the lemon zest, lemon juice, and olive oil in a large bowl. Mix well. Add the arugula and the goji berries and toss. Serve immediately with the soufflé.

(SOUFFLÉ AND SALAD) 460 CALORIES, 20 G PROTEIN, 18 G FAT (5 G SATURATED), 58 G CARBO-HYDRATES, 9 G FIBER, 627 MG SODIUM

CRISPY PUMPKIN SEEDS FALAFEL

SERVES 4 (makes 12 falafel) • SUPERFOODS: Broccoli, Oats, Olive Oil, Pumpkin Seeds

Middle Eastern fare is famous for its filling mix of fiber and heart-healthy fats, but these crunchy fritters go an extra slimming step by ditching the deep fryer and adding magnesium (in the pumpkin seeds), which helps regulate blood sugar.

1 head broccoli, florets only
1/2 cup uncooked old-fashioned oats
2 tablespoons pumpkin seeds
1 teaspoon baking powder

1 15-ounce can chickpeas, drained and rinsed
1/4 cup fresh cilantro
1 teaspoon cumin
2 tablespoons olive oil, divided

FOR THE DRESSING:

1 lemon, zested and juiced
2 tablespoons sesame tahini
2 tablespoons water
1/2 teaspoon dried oregano

2 cups baby spinach
1 large cucumber
4 large (6-inch) whole-wheat pitas

Place the broccoli, oats, pumpkin seeds, and baking powder in a food processor and pulse about twenty times, until finely chopped. Add the chickpeas, cilantro, and cumin. Pulse until it becomes a chunky mixture. Form into twelve, 4-inch-wide falafel patties and transfer to a plate. Refrigerate for 30 minutes.

Heat two large skillets over medium-high heat. Add 1 tablespoon of olive oil to each skillet. Add falafels to each skillet and cook, 8 to 10 minutes, turning several times, until both sides are golden and the falafels are hot.

PREPARE THE DRESSING:

Place the lemon zest and juice, tahini, water, and oregano in a large bowl. Whisk until smooth. Tuck the spinach, cucumber, and three falafels into each pita. Drizzle with the dressing. Serve immediately.

THE DISH (1 PITA WITH 3 FALAFEL) 457 CALORIES, 19 G PROTEIN, 18 G FAT (2 G SATURATED), 64 G CARBOHYDRATES, 15 G FIBER, 756 MG SODIUM

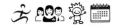

PESTO PASTA SALAD WITH CHERRY TOMATO, TARRAGON, SHALLOTS, AND GRILLED WILD SALMON

SERVES 4 • SUPERFOODS: Olive Oil, Parmesan, Pumpkin Seeds, Whole-Grain Pasta, Wild Salmon

Bring this twist on the potluck staple to your next party. Tarragon, garlic, and shallots pump up the flavor, while omega-3s, protein, and calcium pump up the fat burning.

2 shallots, quartered

Olive oil cooking spray

1 teaspoon sugar

1/2 teaspoon salt, divided

1/2 cup packed tarragon leaves

1/2 cup grated Parmesan

1/4 cup pumpkin seeds

2 tablespoons olive oil

2 garlic cloves, quartered

6 ounces dry, whole-wheat pasta, such as penne or rigatoni, cooked according to the package instructions

1 pint (about 16 ounces) cherry tomatoes, quartered

1 10-ounce wild salmon fillet, skin on

Heat a grill over medium heat. Coat the shallots with cooking spray and sprinkle them with the sugar and half the salt. Place the shallots on the grill and cook about 15 minutes, turning often, until they are well browned and soft. Let cool slightly before chopping.

Place the tarragon leaves, Parmesan, pumpkin seeds, olive oil, garlic, and remaining salt in a mini chopper or pestle. Chop or grind until a chunky pesto forms. Transfer to a large bowl. Add the cooked pasta and cherry tomatoes and mix well.

Coat the salmon with cooking spray and place it on the grill. Cook 6 to 8 minutes, turning once or twice, until the fish is pink in the center but no longer translucent. Transfer to a cutting board. Remove the skin. Using a fork, flake the salmon meat and transfer it to the bowl with the pasta. Add the shallots and toss gently. Serve immediately.

448 CALORIES, 29 G PROTEIN, 19 G FAT (4 G SATURATED), 43 G CARBOHYDRATES, 6 G FIBER, 488 MG SODIUM

CHEF'S NOTE:

Buying fresh tarragon? Look for long, silvery green leaves that are free of blemishes. To separate leaves from stems, turn upside down, pinch the stem between two fingers, and gently slide them down to the tip.

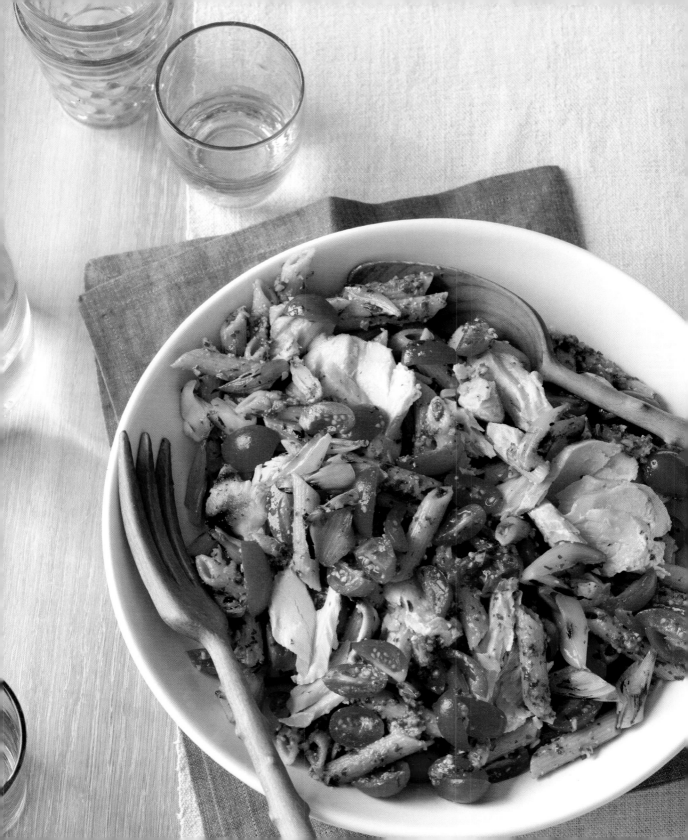

BEEFY NOODLE BOWL WITH KALE, MUSHROOMS, AND BOK CHOY

SERVES 4 • SUPERFOODS: Kale, Mushrooms, Olive Oil, Steak

Slices of juicy beef, hearty noodles, and veggies in a steamy, savory broth—you'll never lift a boring spoonful! You'll also take in fat-targeting vitamin C.

1 ounce dried mushrooms

2 cups boiling water

2 tablespoons light olive oil, divided

12 ounces filet mignon tips or flank steak, thinly sliced

5 ounces mushrooms, chopped

4 garlic cloves, thinly sliced

1 tablespoon peeled, sliced gingerroot

4 cups chopped bok choy (about 8 large leaves)

2 cups chopped kale (about 4 large leaves)

1 15-ounce can reduced-sodium beef broth

1 tablespoon reduced-sodium soy sauce

6 ounces dry buckwheat soba noodles, cooked according
    to the package instructions

$^1/_2$ red bell pepper, thinly sliced

4 scallions, white and green parts, thinly sliced

Rinse the dried mushrooms in a colander under cold running water. Place them in a bowl, add 2 cups boiling water, and soak for 20 minutes. (Do not discard the liquid.)

Heat a large stockpot over medium-high heat. Add 1 tablespoon of the oil and the beef. Cook the beef 1 to 2 minutes, until it browns but is still pink. Transfer to a plate.

Add the remaining oil and the fresh mushrooms, garlic, and ginger. Cook 2 to 3 minutes, stirring often, until the mushrooms soften. Add the bok choy, kale, beef broth, the soaked mushrooms along with their liquid, the soy sauce, and the noodles. Bring to a simmer over medium heat and cook 1 to 2 minutes, scraping up bits that stick to the pan. When the bok choy and kale have softened, add the beef and turn off the heat. Remove the ginger slices and discard. Garnish with the red bell pepper and scallions and serve.

THE DISH

437 CALORIES, 31 G PROTEIN, 15 G FAT (4 G SATURATED), 50 G CARBOHYDRATES, 6 G FIBER, 626 MG SODIUM

PESTO EGG SALAD SANDWICH

SERVES 4 • SUPERFOODS: Artichokes, Eggs, Yogurt

This lighter take on the classic sammie pairs up mayo with just-as-creamy yogurt and adds chunky artichokes and fresh herbs. You'll fill up on protein, fiber, and flavor.

    8 eggs
    6 ounces artichoke hearts (1 cup), chopped
    ½ cup light mayonnaise
    ½ cup plain low-fat yogurt
    1 teaspoon Dijon mustard
    1 teaspoon hot sauce
    ½ cup chopped basil
    ½ cup chopped chives
    4 whole-wheat wraps

Place the eggs in a small saucepan. Cover completely with cold water and bring to a boil over high heat. Turn the heat off and rest, covered, for 15 minutes. Rinse the eggs under cold running water. Crack the eggs and discard the shells.

Chop the eggs and place in a large bowl. Add the artichokes, mayonnaise, yogurt, mustard, hot sauce, basil, and chives. Gently fold the mixture together until the mayonnaise evenly coats the eggs.

Spoon ½ cup of the filling in the center of each wrap. Roll up and serve immediately or wrap in plastic wrap and refrigerate up to 4 hours, until ready to serve.

 448 CALORIES, 23 G PROTEIN, 25 G FAT (5 G SATURATED), 36 G CARBOHYDRATES, 8 G FIBER, 1,089 MG SODIUM

CHEF'S NOTE:
Try this eggy filling for breakfast by serving it warm on whole-grain toast. With a hefty 20 g of protein, it helps jump-start your metabolism for the day.

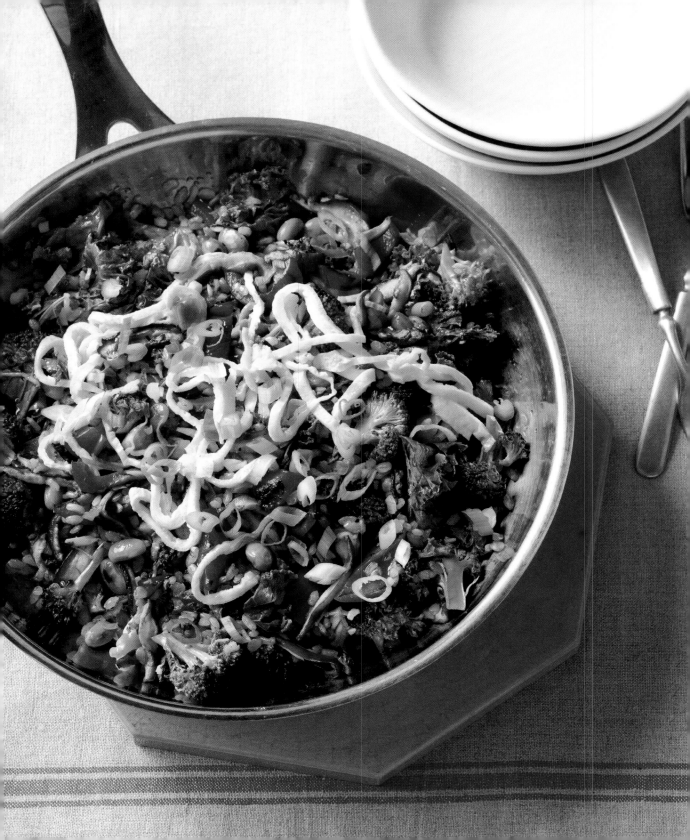

EDAMAME FRIED RICE

SERVES 4 • SUPERFOODS: Broccoli, Edamame, Eggs, Kale, Mushrooms, Olive Oil

Step away from the take-out menu! This dish delivers weight loss by calling on supersatiating soy protein, nutritious veggies, and whole-grain brown rice, which all help keep your blood sugar and insulin levels steady—and your body burning calories.

Olive oil cooking spray

2 eggs, beaten

2 tablespoons light olive oil, divided

8 ounces shiitake mushroom caps, thinly sliced

1 red bell pepper, seeded and chopped

4 cups broccoli florets

4 ounces kale, chopped (about 2 cups)

4 garlic cloves, minced

1 2-inch piece fresh gingerroot, minced (about 2 tablespoons)

1 cup uncooked short-grain brown rice, cooked according to the package instructions

1 1/2 cups frozen, shelled edamame, defrosted

3 tablespoons reduced-sodium soy sauce

2 scallions, thinly sliced

Heat a large skillet over high heat. Remove from the heat and coat with cooking spray. Return the skillet to the burner and add the eggs, turning the pan to coat it with a thin layer of eggs. Cook 30 seconds, loosening the inside edges of the eggs with a spatula. Gently flip the eggs over and cook 10 to 15 seconds. Transfer the eggs to a cutting board.

Heat the same skillet over medium heat. Add half the oil. Add the mushrooms, bell pepper, broccoli, and kale. Cook 4 to 5 minutes, turning often, until the vegetables soften. Add the garlic and ginger. Cook 1 minute, until it becomes fragrant.

Increase the heat to high. Push the vegetables to one side of the skillet and add the remaining olive oil, and the rice. Cook 1 to 2 minutes, turning the rice over with a metal spatula and scraping up bits that stick to the pan. Add the edamame and soy sauce and remove from the heat. Stir two or three times to mix in the soy sauce.

Thinly slice the eggs. Top the rice mixture with the eggs and scallions and serve.

 THE DISH 444 CALORIES, 21 G PROTEIN, 15 G FAT (3 G SATURATED), 62 G CARBOHYDRATES, 9 G FIBER, 517 MG SODIUM

MEXICAN LENTIL WRAPS

SERVES 4 • SUPERFOODS: Avocado, Lentils

The fiber and protein in lentils make them a filling, but skinny, stand-in for beef. In fact, you'll shave off more than 6 grams of saturated fat compared with a loaded fast-food burrito! This one can be speedy, too: Make it the night before, roll in aluminum foil, and stash in the fridge. Lunch, done!

1/4 cup light mayonnaise

1 ounce chipotle chiles en adobo, chopped

1 lime, zested and juiced (about 1/4 cup juice)

1 tablespoon tomato paste

1 teaspoon granulated sugar

1/2 cup dry lentils, cooked according to the package directions

2 cups corn kernels, fresh or frozen (about two large cobs)

1 small cucumber, roughly chopped

1 avocado, cubed

1/4 cup packed cilantro leaves, chopped

1/2 small red onion, minced

4 10-inch whole-wheat wraps

Place the mayonnaise, chiles en adobo, lime zest and juice, tomato paste, and sugar in a blender or mini chopper. Blend until smooth. Transfer to a large bowl. Add the lentils, corn, cucumber, avocado, cilantro, and red onion. Toss to coat.

Set out the four wraps. Spoon a quarter of the mixture onto each wrap. Fold in the edges and roll up. Serve immediately or store filling, refrigerated, for up to two days.

434 CALORIES, 16 G PROTEIN, 15 G FAT (2 G SATURATED), 69 G CARBOHYDRATES, 12 G FIBER, 688 MG SODIUM

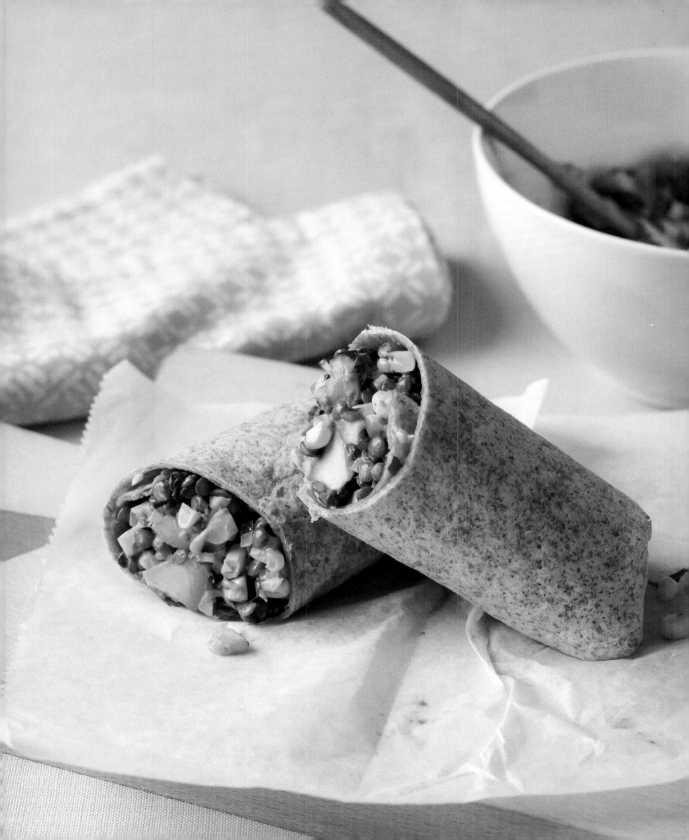

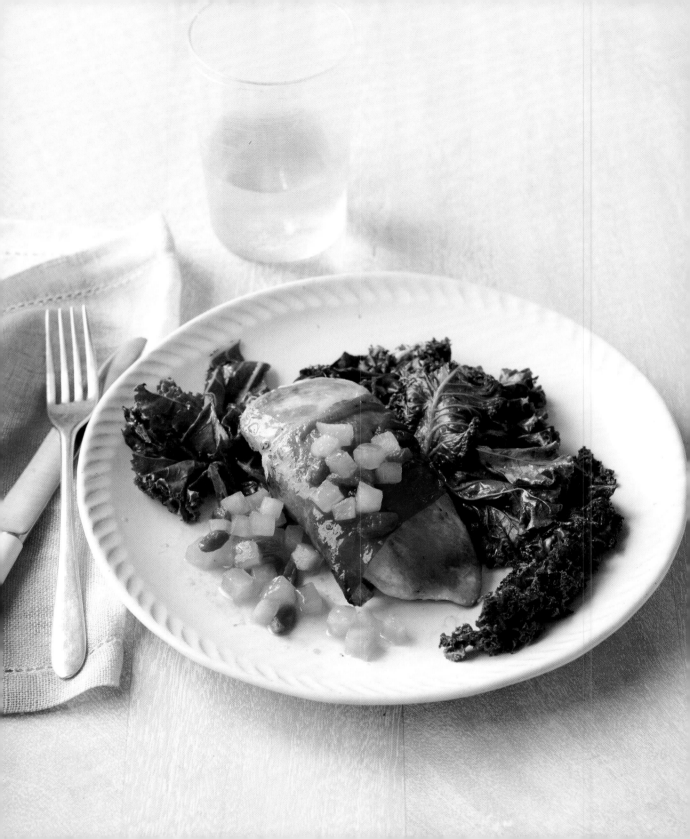

PROSCIUTTO-WRAPPED CHICKEN WITH GINGERED APPLE GOJI CHUTNEY

SERVES 4 • SUPERFOODS: Apples, Goji Berries, Kale, Olive Oil

Nothing says "I'm not dieting" more than bacon! Here, prosciutto fills the role, and chicken is smothered in a sweet, tangy sauce you'll want to lick off the plate.

1 apple, such as Gala or Golden Delicious, cored, peeled,
     and chopped
$1/4$ cup goji berries
2 teaspoons grated fresh gingerroot
2 tablespoons brown sugar
2 tablespoons cider vinegar or rice wine vinegar
$1/8$ teaspoon salt
4 large boneless, skinless chicken breasts (6 ounces
     each), trimmed of excess fat
4 slices prosciutto, trimmed of excess fat
2 tablespoons olive oil, divided
1 large bunch kale (about 10 ounces), chopped

In a small saucepan, place the apple, goji berries, ginger, brown sugar, vinegar, and salt. Bring to a boil, then reduce to a simmer and cook about 20 minutes, until most of the liquid has evaporated and a thick chutney starts to form. Remove from the heat and set aside.

Heat the oven to 400°F. Wrap each chicken breast in one slice of prosciutto. Heat a large, oven-safe skillet over medium-high heat. Add 1 tablespoon of the olive oil. Add the chicken breasts and cook 1 minute, turning once to brown the prosciutto. Transfer to the oven and bake 10 minutes, or until the chicken is cooked through.

In a second large, oven-safe skillet, warm the remaining olive oil over medium heat. Add the kale and cook 1 to 2 minutes, turning often, until the kale starts to soften. Slide the skillet into the oven and bake 5 minutes, or until the kale starts to crisp. Remove both skillets from the oven and place the chicken and kale on plates. Top with chutney and serve immediately.

474 CALORIES, 60 G PROTEIN, 15 G FAT (3 G SATURATED), 23 G CARBOHYDRATES, 3 G FIBER, 622 MG SODIUM

LENTIL NACHOS WITH CHEESE AND AVOCADO

SERVES 4 • SUPERFOODS: Avocado, Lentils, Mushrooms, Olive Oil

Lentils often get pigeonholed as side dishes or in soups, but here they take scrumptious center stage as the fiber- and protein-packed base of this irresistibly cheesy dip.

2 teaspoons olive oil

1 medium red or yellow onion, minced

5 ounces mushrooms, such as cremini or white button, finely chopped, stems included

1 small jalapeño, chopped

1 cup dry red or brown lentils, rinsed well under cold running water

1 tablespoon taco seasoning

2 1/2 cups water

3/4 cup grated Colby or pepper jack cheese (3 ounces)

1/2 ripe avocado, cut into 1-inch cubes

4 ounces whole-grain or whole-wheat pita chips (about 24 chips)

Heat a large skillet over medium-high heat. Add the olive oil, onion, mushrooms, and jalapeño. Cook 2 to 3 minutes, stirring often, until the onion softens. Add the lentils and the taco seasoning and cook 1 minute, until the spices become fragrant. Add the water. Cover and reduce the heat to low. Simmer, covered, 15 to 20 minutes, until the lentils are soft and the liquid is absorbed. Turn off the heat.

Sprinkle cheese over the lentils and cover for 30 seconds, or until the cheese melts. Top with avocado cubes. Serve immediately with the pita chips.

 THE DISH (LENTILS PLUS 8 PITA CHIPS) 474 CALORIES, 23 G PROTEIN, 17 G FAT (6 G SATURATED), 57 G CARBOHYDRATES, 18 G FIBER, 451 MG SODIUM

COOL SHRIMP SALAD WITH QUINOA, GRAPEFRUIT, AND AVOCADO

SERVES 4 • SUPERFOODS: Avocado, Olive Oil, Pomegranate, Quinoa, Yogurt

With only 5 calories per piece and plenty of protein, shrimp is an honorary Drop 10 superfood. It brings its calorie-torching strength to the next level by joining forces with quinoa and yogurt to smack down fat with 23 g of metabolism-revving protein per serving.

$1/4$ cup plain, low-fat yogurt

2 tablespoons honey

2 teaspoons Dijon mustard

2 tablespoons olive oil

$1/4$ cup chopped chives

1 pound cooked, chilled shrimp, tails removed

1 cup cooked quinoa

1 Hass avocado, sliced

2 pink grapefruits, sectioned

1 cup pomegranate seeds

4 cups baby spinach leaves

In a small bowl, whisk together the yogurt, honey, mustard, olive oil, and chives until smooth. Set aside.

Place the shrimp, quinoa, avocado, grapefruits, pomegranate seeds, and spinach in a large bowl and toss gently. Transfer to a platter and drizzle with the dressing. Serve immediately.

 THE DISH 433 CALORIES, 23 G PROTEIN, 15 G FAT (2 G SATURATED), 52 G CARBOHYDRATES, 10 G FIBER, 760 MG SODIUM

CHEF'S NOTE:
Keep precooked shrimp in your freezer and add them to salads
and pastas to bump up the protein count. To thaw, place them
in a colander and rinse under cold running water.

PASTA PUTTANESCA

SERVES 4 • SUPERFOODS: Parmesan, Olive Oil, Sardines, Whole-Grain Pasta

The Mediterranean style of eating is famously healthy and naturally slimming, thanks to omega-3s, fiber, veggies, and olive oil—which come together in this pretty pasta. *Mangia!*

12 ounces dry whole-wheat spaghetti or linguine

2 tablespoons extra-virgin olive oil

4 garlic cloves, thinly sliced

1/4 teaspoon crushed red pepper

1 tablespoon capers, drained and chopped

1/2 cup olives, such as Kalamata or Cerignola, pitted and roughly chopped

1 28-ounce can diced tomatoes

1 canned sardine, packed in water, rinsed

1/2 cup shaved Parmesan

2 basil sprigs, stem removed, leaves torn

Cook the pasta according to the package instructions. Turn off the heat. Drain the pasta, reserving 1/2 cup of cooking water, and return the pasta to the pot.

Meanwhile, heat the olive oil in a large skillet over medium heat. Add the garlic and red pepper and cook 1 to 2 minutes, stirring, until garlic is slightly toasted. Add the capers and olives and cook 2 minutes. Add the tomatoes, along with the juice they are packed in. Cook about 2 minutes, until the mixture thickens. Add the sardine, breaking it up with a fork. Add the pasta and toss to coat. Garnish with the Parmesan and basil and serve immediately.

THE DISH

468 CALORIES, 19 G PROTEIN, 13 G FAT (3 G SATURATED), 74 G CARBOHYDRATES, 9 G FIBER, 769 MG SODIUM

CHEF'S NOTE:
Canned, diced tomatoes can be high in bloating sodium, so check labels and pick a brand with less than 270 mg sodium per 1/2-cup serving.

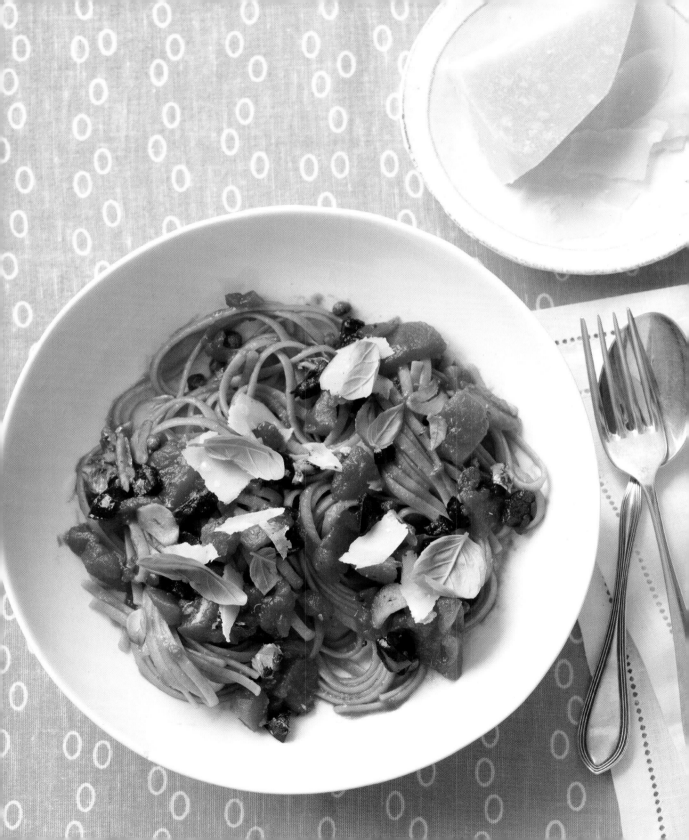

CURRY CHICKEN SALAD SANDWICH

SERVES 4 • SUPERFOODS: Apples, Cherries, Edamame, Yogurt

Tart apples and sweet dried cherries are bright spots in this creamy, somewhat spicy recipe. You'll feel spoiled (by the fancy flavors), satiated (by the filling fiber and protein), and smaller (you get all this for under 500 calories!).

2 boneless, skinless chicken breasts (6 ounces each)

2 teaspoons curry powder

1/4 teaspoon salt

Olive oil cooking spray

1 Granny Smith apple, cored, diced (about 1 1/2 apples)

1/2 cup frozen, shelled edamame, defrosted

1/3 cup dried cherries

1/2 cup light mayonnaise

1/2 plain low-fat Greek yogurt

8 slices whole-grain sandwich bread

Heat the oven to 400°F. Sprinkle each chicken breast with 1 teaspoon of the curry powder and the salt.

Heat a small skillet over high heat. Remove the skillet from the heat, coat it with cooking spray, and return it to the stove. Add the chicken and cook 2 to 3 minutes, turning once, until the chicken is browned. Slide the skillet into the oven and bake 6 to 8 minutes, until the chicken is cooked through and no longer pink in the center. Transfer to a cutting board and allow to rest 5 minutes before slicing into 1/2-inch cubes.

Transfer the chicken to a large bowl. Add the apple, edamame, dried cherries, mayonnaise, and yogurt. Gently fold the mixture and place 1/2 cup of the filling on each of four slices of bread. Top each with a second slice and serve.

453 CALORIES, 29 G PROTEIN, 10 G FAT (1 G SATURATED), 58 G CARBOHYDRATES, 8 G FIBER, 714 MG SODIUM

CHEF'S NOTE:
Make this salad up to 3 days ahead to bring to picnics or potlucks,
or simply to keep on hand for family lunch bags.

SWEET POTATO SKINS WITH BROCCOLI AND PEPPER JACK CHEESE

SERVES 4 • SUPERFOODS: Broccoli, Olive Oil, Peanuts, Sweet Potatoes, Yogurt

Loaded spuds aren't only for happy hour: Nutritious and filling enough for a meal, our take gives you the flavor you want, with a dose of vitamin C, healthy oils, and resistant starch to help you burn excess fat.

4 large sweet potatoes, each cut into 4 wedges
Olive oil cooking spray
2 slices nitrate-free turkey bacon
1 tablespoon olive oil
4 cups broccoli florets
1/4 teaspoon salt

1/2 cup water
3/4 cup grated pepper jack cheese (3 ounces)
1/2 cup plain low-fat yogurt
2 scallions, white and green parts, thinly sliced
1/4 cup unsalted peanuts, chopped

Heat the oven to 400°F. Place the potato wedges on a baking sheet and coat with cooking spray. Bake 45 to 50 minutes, until the wedges are soft. Coat another baking sheet with cooking spray. Place the bacon on it and bake 10 to 15 minutes, until crisp. Transfer to a cutting board and chop. Set aside.

Heat a large skillet over high heat. Add the olive oil, broccoli, and salt. Cook 4 to 5 minutes, stirring often, until the broccoli softens. Add 1/2 cup of water and cover. Cook 1 minute, until the broccoli is fork-tender.

Place the broccoli in a bowl. Scoop out the flesh from the potato wedges and add it to the broccoli. (Do not discard the potato skins.) Add the cheese and stir to combine.

Place the potato skins back on the baking sheet. Spoon the broccoli mixture into the skins and bake for 35 to 40 minutes, until the centers are soft.

Place the yogurt and the scallions in a small bowl. Stir well. Set out four plates and place four potato skins on each. Garnish with the yogurt-scallion mixture, bacon, and peanuts and serve.

THE DISH (4 POTATO SKINS, LOADED) 421 CALORIES, 16 G PROTEIN, 11 G FAT (3 G SATURATED), 67 G CARBOHYDRATES, 12 G FIBER, 478 MG SODIUM

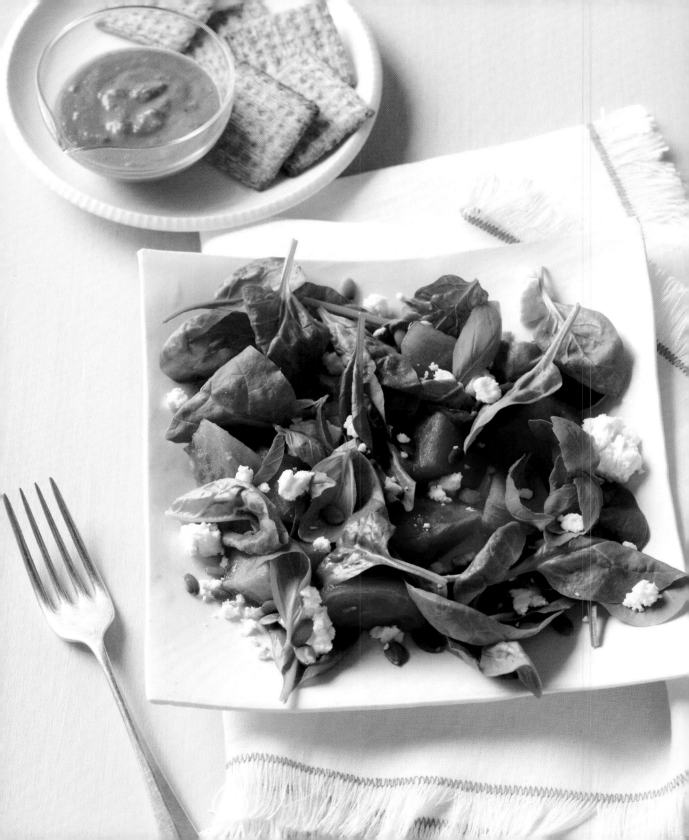

BABY SPINACH AND WATERMELON SALAD WITH CREAMY GOJI DRESSING

SERVES 4 • SUPERFOODS: Goji Berries, Olive Oil, Parmesan, Pumpkin Seeds

We know what you're thinking, but give these unusual flavor matches a chance. Like a great mashup, they make beautiful music together—and chime in with more than half your daily dose of fat-burning vitamin C and all the vision-protecting A you need.

> 6 tablespoons boiling water
>
> 2 tablespoons goji berries
>
> 1 tablespoon tomato paste
>
> 1/4 cup grated Parmesan
>
> 1/2 teaspoon dried oregano
>
> 1 tablespoon olive oil
>
> 10 ounces baby spinach (about 8 cups)
>
> 4 cups cubed watermelon
>
> 1 cup crumbled feta cheese
>
> 1/2 cup pumpkin seeds
>
> 1/2 cup fresh basil leaves
>
> 24 whole-wheat crackers, such as Triscuits

Place the water in a small bowl and add the goji berries. Allow to rest for 5 minutes, or until the berries plump up and the water cools slightly.

Transfer the berries, along with any remaining water, to a blender. Add the tomato paste, Parmesan, oregano, and olive oil. Blend until smooth. Set aside in a small bowl.

Arrange the spinach on a large platter. Top with the watermelon. Sprinkle with the feta cheese and pumpkin seeds. Drizzle with the dressing (save some to dip crackers) and garnish with basil leaves. Serve immediately with the crackers.

THE DISH (SALAD PLUS 6 CRACKERS) 446 CALORIES, 22 G PROTEIN, 25 G FAT (8 G SATURATED), 41 G CARBOHYDRATES, 7 G FIBER, 723 MG SODIUM

SPICY CHICKEN CLUB WITH LEMONY MAYO SPREAD

SERVES 4 • SUPERFOODS: Artichokes, Olive Oil, Parmesan, Yogurt

Strained, low-fat Greek yogurt makes the perfect creamy swap for some of the mayo or sour cream in any recipe. You'll save fat and calories, but gain protein to spark your metabolism. The flavor? Every bit as yummy.

2 boneless, skinless chicken
   breasts (6 ounces each)
1/2 teaspoon cayenne powder
1/4 teaspoon freshly ground black
   pepper
2 teaspoons extra-virgin olive oil
1/3 cup grated Parmesan
1/3 cup artichoke hearts, chopped
   (about 3 ounces)
3 tablespoons light mayonnaise

2 tablespoons plain low-fat
   Greek yogurt
1 lemon, zested and juiced
1 whole-wheat baguette
   (12 ounces), cut into four equal
   pieces
2 cups baby spinach or mesclun
   greens
1/4 cup fresh basil leaves

Heat the oven to 400°F. Sprinkle the chicken with cayenne and black pepper. Heat a medium oven-safe skillet over medium heat. Add the olive oil and chicken and cook 3 to 4 minutes, without turning, until the chicken turns golden. Turn and cook 2 to 3 minutes, until it starts to brown.

Slide the skillet into the oven and cook 6 to 8 minutes, until the chicken is cooked through and no longer pink in the center. Transfer chicken to a cutting board.

In a small bowl, combine the Parmesan, artichokes, mayonnaise, yogurt, and lemon zest and juice. Stir well to combine.

Cut each chicken breast diagonally, against the grain, into eight thin slices. Slice each piece of baguette horizontally into three thin slices. Layer 1 slice of chicken, a few leaves of the spinach or mesclun, and the basil on the bottom slice. Top with a heaping tablespoon of the artichoke mixture. Repeat with next layer and top with last piece of baguette. Serve immediately or wrap in plastic wrap and refrigerate until ready to serve.

(1 SANDWICH) 467 CALORIES, 41 G PROTEIN, 12 G FAT (2 G SATURATED), 52 G CARBOHYDRATES, 7 G FIBER, 886 MG SODIUM

HERITAGE PEANUT SOUP

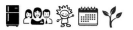

SERVES 4 • SUPERFOODS: Apples, Olive Oil, Peanuts

While this rich and chunky soup will leave you warm and cozy on a cool day, its haul of protein (from the peanuts and chicken) lights a fire under your metabolism, helping you double your calorie burn as you digest all the deliciousness.

3 skinless, boneless chicken
   breasts (about 6 ounces each)
$1/4$ teaspoon salt
$1/4$ teaspoon cayenne pepper or
   1 teaspoon mild ground red
   pepper
1 teaspoon fresh thyme leaves
1 tablespoon light olive oil
1 red onion, chopped
1 apple, peeled, cored, chopped

$1/2$ cup dry-roasted unsalted
   peanuts, plus 2 tablespoons,
   chopped, for garnish
2 garlic cloves, minced
1 tablespoon tomato paste
3 cups water
1 15-ounce can diced tomatoes
4 scallions, white and green parts,
   thinly sliced
24 whole-wheat crackers

Sprinkle the chicken with the salt, cayenne or ground red pepper, and thyme. Heat a large stockpot over medium heat. Add the olive oil and the chicken. Cook 3 to 4 minutes, turning the breasts once or twice, until they brown on both sides. Transfer the chicken to a plate.

In the same stockpot, add the onion, apple, $1/2$ cup peanuts, and garlic. Cook 3 to 4 minutes, stirring occasionally, until the onion starts to soften. Add the tomato paste and reduce the heat to low. Cook 1 minute, stirring constantly, until the paste becomes fragrant. Add the water and diced tomatoes, along with their juices.

Return the chicken to the pot and bring to a steady simmer over medium heat. Cover and cook 20 to 25 minutes, or until the chicken is cooked through. Remove the chicken and cool 5 minutes.

Blend the soup, using an immersion blender (or carefully transfer to a food processor in batches). Shred the chicken and return it to the soup. Divide the soup among four bowls and garnish with scallions and remaining peanuts. Serve with crackers.

(SOUP, PLUS 6 WHOLE-WHEAT CRACKERS) 450 CALORIES, 34 G PROTEIN, 20 G FAT (2 G SATU-RATED), 34 G CARBOHYDRATES, 6 G FIBER, 706 MG SODIUM

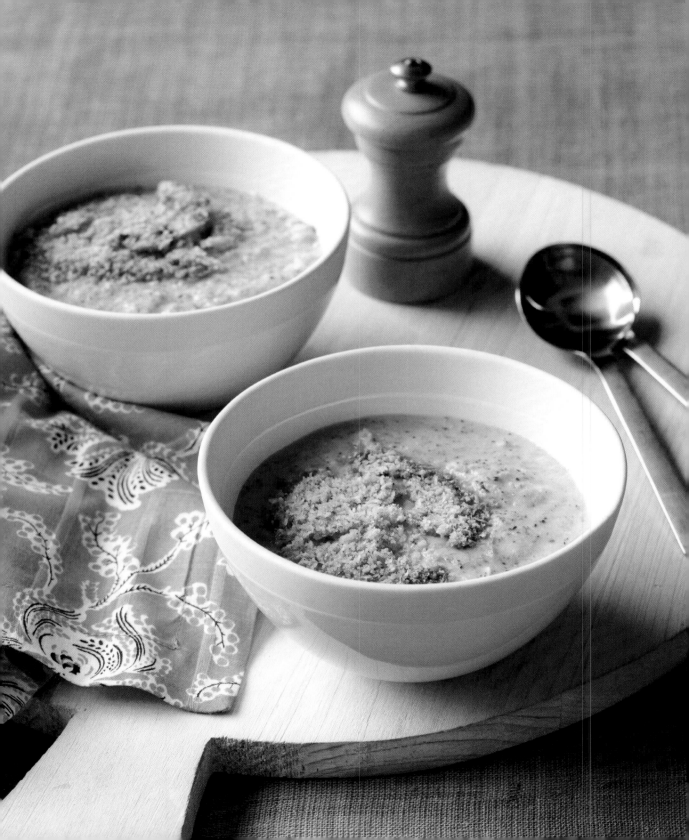

CREAM OF BROCCOLI SOUP WITH PARMESAN CROUTONS

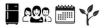

SERVES 4 • SUPERFOODS: Broccoli, Edamame, Olive Oil, Parmesan

One taste and you'll wonder how something this indulgent can help you lose weight and be healthier. Potatoes are the creamy secret here, and the edamame ups the level of pound-peeling protein.

1 tablespoon olive oil

1 head broccoli, top cut into florets, stalk peeled and finely chopped

1/2 small white onion

1 teaspoon curry powder

1 white potato (about 6 ounces), peeled and diced

1 cup frozen shelled edamame, thawed

1 15-ounce can reduced-sodium chicken broth

3/4 cup half-and-half

CROUTONS:

Olive oil cooking spray

1/2 cup grated Parmesan

2 tablespoons Italian bread crumbs

Heat a large stockpot over medium-high heat. Add the olive oil, broccoli stalk, onion, and curry powder. Cook 3 to 4 minutes, stirring often, until the onion begins to soften. Add the potato, edamame, and chicken broth. Bring to a simmer over medium heat. Reduce the heat to low and simmer, covered, 20 minutes, until the potato is soft. Add the broccoli florets and half-and-half and simmer 10 minutes, until the florets are soft. Blend the soup in a blender or food processor until smooth. Serve immediately with croutons.

PREPARE THE CROUTONS:

Heat the oven to 400°F. Coat a large cookie sheet with cooking spray. In a small bowl, mix together the Parmesan and bread crumbs. Place 8 heaping teaspoons of the Parmesan mixture onto the baking sheet, spaced 2 inches apart. Bake 2 to 3 minutes, until the edges brown. Remove the croutons from the oven and allow to cool on the baking sheet.

(SOUP, PLUS 2 CROUTONS) 368 CALORIES, 20 G PROTEIN, 15 G FAT (6 G SATURATED), 42 G CARBOHYDRATES, 5 G FIBER, 783 MG SODIUM

HOT AND SOUR SOUP

SERVES 4 • SUPERFOODS: Eggs, Mushrooms, Olive Oil

Whoever decided soup belongs on the appetizer menu never made one like this. Pork, tofu, eggs, soba noodles—one bowl has almost as much protein power as two servings of steak! That will get you about halfway to your daily goal and all the way to your next meal minus hunger pangs.

1 14-ounce package extra-firm tofu

3 tablespoons rice vinegar

2 tablespoons reduced-sodium soy sauce

2 tablespoons cornstarch

1 tablespoon red chili paste, such as sambal

1 teaspoon granulated sugar

2 cups dried mushrooms (2 ounces), such as wood ears
    or shiitake

1 cup boiling water

1 pork chop (12 ounces), excess fat trimmed

1 tablespoon light olive oil

8 ounces shiitake mushrooms, stems discarded, caps
    thinly sliced

1 1-inch piece fresh gingerroot, peeled and grated (about
    1 tablespoon)

2 cups reduced-sodium chicken broth

1 8-ounce can bamboo shoots

1 cup warm water

1 large egg, lightly beaten

4 scallions, green and white parts, thinly sliced

4 ounces soba noodles, cooked according to the package
    instructions

Place a strainer in the sink. Add the tofu. Place a heavy saucepan on top of the tofu. Allow it to rest for at least 1 hour, until the tofu shrinks by half. Cut into 1-inch cubes and set aside.

    Meanwhile, combine the rice vinegar, soy sauce, cornstarch, chili paste, and sugar in a medium bowl. Whisk well and set aside.

Rinse the dried mushrooms under cold running water to remove any dirt. Place them in a small bowl with the boiling water and let rest for 15 minutes.

Cut the meat from the pork chop and reserve the bone. Slice the meat into thin, $\frac{1}{8}$-inch strips and set aside. In a stockpot, heat the oil over medium heat. Add the fresh mushrooms and bone and cook over medium heat, stirring occasionally, until the bone and the mushrooms are browned. Add the sliced pork and cook 2 to 3 minutes, stirring occasionally, until the pork browns. Add the ginger. Cook 1 minute, stirring often, until the ginger becomes fragrant. Discard the bone.

Add the tofu, soaked mushrooms along with their liquid, chicken broth, bamboo shoots, and warm water. Bring to a simmer over medium-low heat. Add the egg and cook 30 seconds, stirring well, until the egg cooks and forms delicate threads throughout the soup.

Stir in the rice vinegar mixture and soba noodles and cook 30 seconds, until the soup thickens. Remove from the heat and garnish with the scallions. Serve immediately.

 433 CALORIES, 40 G PROTEIN, 11 G FAT (3 G SATURATED), 45 G CARBOHYDRATES, 10 G FIBER, 831 MG SODIUM

BEEF BARLEY

SERVES 4 • SUPERFOODS: Mushrooms, Oats, Olive Oil, Steak

Warm up while guarding against cold bugs! Not only does the protein in beef crank up your calorie burn, but its easy-to-absorb iron strengthens your immune system. Plus, barley contains beta-glucan, a type of fiber that helps you shrink and builds your body's defenses against infection.

2 tablespoons olive oil, divided
1 large red onion, chopped
4 carrots, peeled and chopped
2 celery stalks, chopped
2 garlic cloves, chopped
1 pound lean beef stew meat
1 tablespoon oat flour
1/2 teaspoon salt
1/4 teaspoon freshly ground black pepper
1 cup tomato puree
10 ounces cremini or white button mushrooms, brushed clean, sliced
1 15-ounce can low-sodium beef broth
4 cups water
1/2 cup uncooked barley
2 dried bay leaves (optional)
2 cups packed baby spinach leaves
1/4 cup chopped fresh flat-leaf parsley
4 teaspoons lemon zest

Heat a large stockpot over high heat. Add half the olive oil, onion, carrots, celery, and garlic. Reduce the heat to medium and cook 5 to 6 minutes, stirring often, until the onion browns slightly and the vegetables start to soften.

Place the beef on a plate and sprinkle with the flour, salt, and pepper. Push the vegetables in the pot to one side and add the remaining olive oil. Add the beef and cook 3 to 4 minutes, stirring occasionally, until the beef begins to brown.

Add the tomato puree and mushrooms. Stir to coat the beef and vegetables. Cook 1 minute. Add the beef broth and 4 cups of water. Add the barley and bay leaves, if using. Bring to a slow boil over high heat, then reduce to low. Cover and simmer about 1 1/2 hours, until the beef is tender and a thick soup has formed. Remove from the heat, stir in the spinach, and cover for 1 minute to allow the spinach to wilt. Garnish with parsley and lemon zest and serve immediately.

THE DISH 429 CALORIES, 36 G PROTEIN, 14 G FAT (3 G SATURATED), 41 G CARBOHYDRATES, 12 G FIBER, 699 MG SODIUM

CHICKEN-FRIED FLANK STEAK OVER CREAMY ARTICHOKES WITH YOGURT AND PARMESAN

SERVES 4 • SUPERFOODS: Artichokes, Broccoli, Eggs, Oats, Olive Oil, Parmesan, Steak, Yogurt

Traditional chicken-fried steak is practically a heart attack on a plate, but this version cooks in a pan with less oil, saving you tons of unwanted calories. The fiber-dense artichokes and creamy yogurt combine to create a killer (tasting, that is!) gravy.

3/4 pound flank steak, trimmed of excess fat

1/2 teaspoon salt

1/2 teaspoon freshly ground black pepper

2 eggs, beaten

1 cup oat flour

3 tablespoons extra-virgin olive oil

Olive oil cooking spray

1 head broccoli, cut into florets, stem discarded

1 teaspoon fresh thyme leaves

1 cup reduced-sodium chicken broth

1 9-ounce package frozen artichoke hearts, defrosted and chopped

1/2 cup plain low-fat Greek yogurt

1/3 cup grated Parmesan

Slice the steak into four equal portions. Using a meat mallet, pound each into a 1-inch-thick steak. Sprinkle with the salt and black pepper. Place the eggs and flour in separate, shallow dishes. Dredge the steaks in the eggs, and then press into the flour.

Heat a large skillet over high heat. Add the oil and the steaks. Reduce the heat to medium and cook 6 to 8 minutes, turning twice, until a golden crust forms and the steaks are pink inside, but no longer red. Set out four plates and place a steak on each.

Coat the same skillet with cooking spray. Heat the skillet over medium heat and add the broccoli and thyme. Cook the broccoli 1 to 2 minutes, stirring often, until it starts to soften. Add the chicken broth and artichokes and cover. Cook 2 minutes, until the broccoli is tender and most of the liquid has evaporated. Turn off the heat. Slowly stir in the yogurt a tablespoon at a time, then stir in the Parmesan. Divide the artichoke mixture among the four plates and serve immediately.

THE DISH 458 CALORIES, 33 G PROTEIN, 24 G FAT (7 G SATURATED), 29 G CARBOHYDRATES, 8 G FIBER, 764 MG SODIUM

VEGGIE PROSCIUTTO PIZZA

SERVES 6 • SUPERFOODS: Artichokes, Mushrooms, Olive Oil, Parmesan

A traditional *quattro stagione* pizza puts a different topping on each quarter of the pie. But by loading up the entire surface with superfoods, plus savory prosciutto, you'll enjoy a heartier slice.

> 16 ounces frozen, whole-wheat pizza dough, defrosted
>
> 1 cup low-sodium jarred pasta sauce
>
> 1 1/2 cups grated part-skim mozzarella
>
> 10 ounces cremini or white button mushrooms, thinly sliced
>
> 4 cups baby spinach, wilted
>
> 1 9-ounce bag frozen artichoke hearts, defrosted, chopped
>
> 1 ounce (about 2 slices) thinly sliced prosciutto, excess fat removed, cut into strips
>
> 3/4 cup grated Parmesan
>
> 1 tablespoon extra-virgin olive oil
>
> 1 teaspoon crushed red pepper

Heat the oven to 400˚F. Roll the pizza dough out into a disk, about 10 inches in diameter. Transfer to a pizza screen or aluminum pizza pan. Spoon on the pasta sauce, and smooth it across the dough with the back of a spoon.

Sprinkle the mozzarella evenly over the surface. Scatter the mushrooms, spinach, artichokes, and prosciutto. Sprinkle the Parmesan over all the toppings. Drizzle on the olive oil and sprinkle with the crushed red pepper.

Bake 15 to 20 minutes, until the edges are brown and the cheese is bubbly. Cool 5 minutes, slice into 6 pieces, and serve.

(1 SLICE) 366 CALORIES, 21 G PROTEIN, 13 G FAT (5 G SATURATED), 43 G CARBOHYDRATES, 5 G FIBER, 814 MG SODIUM

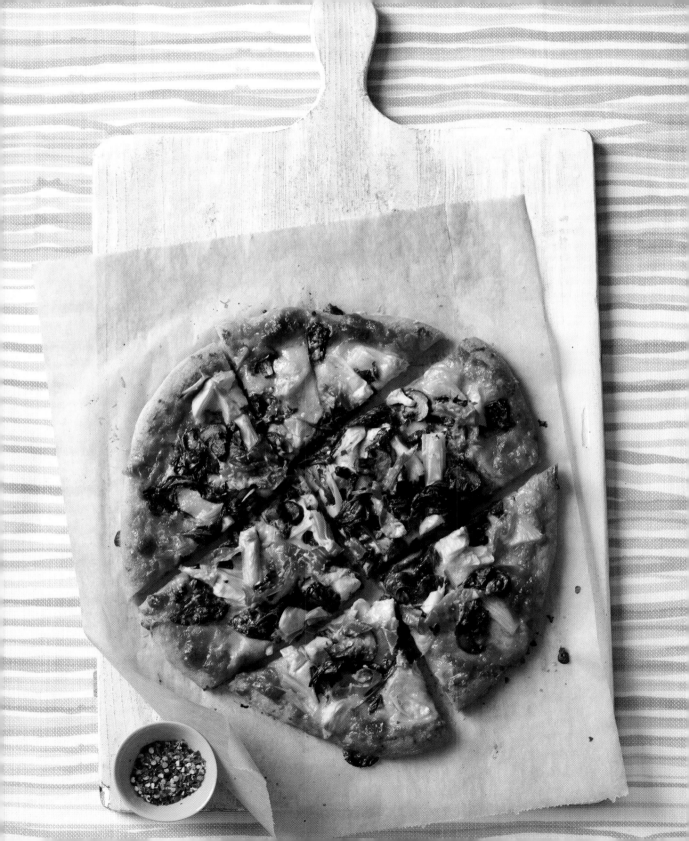

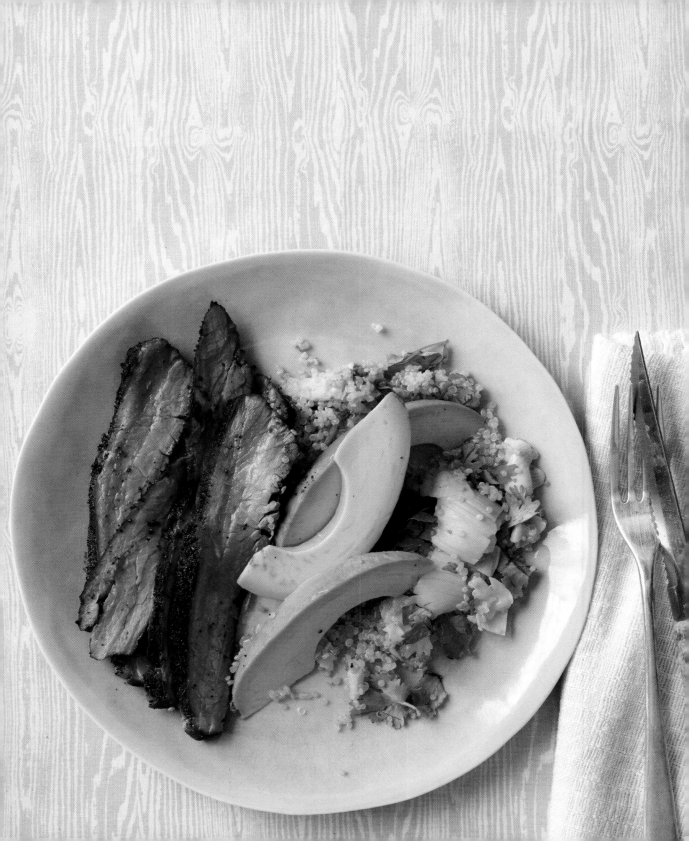

COFFEE CHILI-RUBBED FLANK STEAK WITH LIME AVOCADO QUINOA

SERVES 4 • SUPERFOODS: Artichoke, Avocado, Coffee, Quinoa, Steak

It's a good thing that steak's protein helps you build muscle—you'll need it to fight over who gets the leftovers! Coffee may seem like an unusual rub ingredient, but it lends the meat a deeply smoky and delicious flavor. Eat leftovers in a salad the next day or use them in the Beefy Breakfast Burrito on page 60 or Steak and Eggs Rancheros on page 78.

$^3/_4$ cup uncooked quinoa

1 $^1/_4$ cups water

1 9-ounce package frozen artichoke hearts, defrosted, roughly chopped

1 Hass avocado, sliced

2 limes, zested and juiced (about $^1/_2$ cup)

$^3/_4$ teaspoon salt, divided

$^1/_2$ cup cilantro, chopped

1 teaspoon mild chili powder

1 teaspoon finely ground coffee

$^1/_2$ teaspoon garlic powder

$^1/_2$ teaspoon ground coriander

$^1/_4$ teaspoon freshly ground black pepper

1 pound flank steak, trimmed of excess fat

Vegetable oil cooking spray

Rinse the quinoa well under cold running water. In a small saucepan, bring 1 $^1/_4$ cups of water to a boil. Add the quinoa and stir well. Reduce the heat to low and simmer, covered, for 8 to 10 minutes, until the quinoa is soft and has tripled in size. Remove from the heat and allow the quinoa to cool in the saucepan for 5 minutes. Add the artichokes, avocado, lime juice and zest, and $^1/_4$ teaspoon salt. Garnish with cilantro.

In a small bowl, place the chili powder, ground coffee, garlic powder, coriander, remaining $^1/_2$ teaspoon of the salt, and the black pepper. Stir to combine. Place the flank steak on a plate and sprinkle both sides with the chili mixture.

Heat a large grill over high heat. Coat both sides of the flank steak with a thin layer of vegetable oil cooking spray. Place it on the grill and cook 10 minutes on each side. Remove from the heat and let rest for 5 minutes before slicing. Serve with the lime avocado quinoa.

THE DISH 465 CALORIES, 34 G PROTEIN, 21 G FAT (5 G SATURATED), 37 G CARBOHYDRATES, 11 G FIBER, 565 MG SODIUM

WARM, STUFFED CAESAR MUSHROOMS

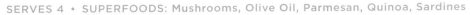

SERVES 4 • SUPERFOODS: Mushrooms, Olive Oil, Parmesan, Quinoa, Sardines

These elegant 'shrooms might remind you of stuffed baked crab, but the slimming superfoods ensure you won't have to stuff yourself into your swimsuit. The omega-3s in the fish might even help you burn more fat at your next workout.

8 medium portobello mushroom caps, brushed clean with
    a damp paper towel
Olive oil cooking spray
2 cups cooked quinoa
2 canned sardines packed in oil, drained
1 lemon, zested and juiced (about $\frac{1}{2}$ cup juice)
1 tablespoon extra-virgin olive oil
1 teaspoon Dijon mustard
1 teaspoon Worcestershire sauce
1 cup grated Parmesan
6 cups shredded romaine lettuce or mesclun greens

Heat oven to 400°F. Line a baking sheet with aluminum foil. Using a spoon, scrape out the black gills from the underside of the mushrooms. Coat both sides of each mushroom with cooking spray. Set them top-side down on the foil.

In a medium bowl, place the quinoa, sardines, lemon zest and juice, olive oil, mustard, and Worcestershire sauce. Mix well. Spoon about $\frac{1}{4}$ cup of the mixture onto each mushroom. Press 2 tablespoons of Parmesan on top of the quinoa filling on each mushroom.

Bake 15 to 20 minutes, or until the tops are golden and the mushrooms are soft. Serve immediately over the greens.

379 CALORIES, 23 G PROTEIN, 20 G FAT (6 G SATURATED), 33 G CARBOHYDRATES, 8 G FIBER, 542 MG SODIUM

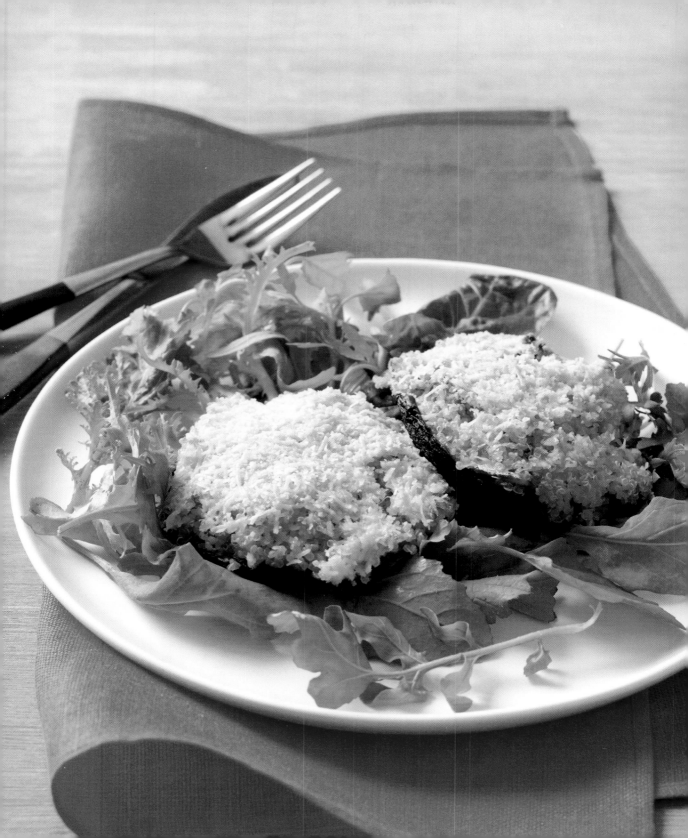

SPAGHETTI POMODORO

SERVES 4 • SUPERFOODS: Olive Oil, Parmesan, Whole-Grain Pasta

Pasta used to be off-limits to dieters, but thankfully that "rule" has been reversed. In fact, up to 65 percent of your daily calories can come from healthy carbs such as whole-wheat noodles! The fiber in them prevents you from absorbing a portion of the fat and calories in your meal.

> 2 tablespoons extra-virgin olive oil
> 1 red bell pepper, seeded, minced
> 4 garlic cloves, thinly sliced
> 1 teaspoon dried or freshly chopped oregano
> 1 28-ounce can diced tomatoes
> 1/2 cup white wine (optional)
> 8 cups baby spinach
> 2 tablespoons water
> 10 ounces whole-wheat spaghetti, cooked according to
>   the package instructions
> 1/2 cup grated Parmesan

Heat a large skillet over medium-low heat. Add the olive oil, bell pepper, garlic, and oregano. Cook 3 to 4 minutes, stirring often, until the pepper softens and the garlic becomes fragrant.

Add the tomatoes, along with their juices, and the white wine (if using). Cook 15 to 20 minutes, stirring occasionally, until the sauce reduces by one-third.

Heat a separate large skillet over high heat and add the spinach with 2 tablespoons of water. Cook 20 to 30 seconds, stirring often, until the spinach wilts but is still bright green. Add it and the cooked pasta to the sauce and toss well. Turn off the heat and sprinkle with Parmesan. Serve immediately.

THE DISH (USING WINE) 457 CALORIES, 19 G PROTEIN, 11 G FAT (3 G SATURATED), 70 G CARBOHYDRATES, 11 G FIBER, 674 MG SODIUM

CHEF'S NOTE:

Despite its lack of meat, this recipe is ultra-filling. If you're craving chewier bites, however, swap out spinach for 2 cups of broccoli, chopped into small florets.

QUINOA-CRUSTED WILD SALMON WITH BROCCOLI COUSCOUS

SERVES 4 • SUPERFOODS: Broccoli, Eggs, Goji Berries, Oats, Olive Oil, Parmesan, Pumpkin Seeds, Quinoa, Whole-Grain Pasta, Wild Salmon

This colorful meal fits a tasty goodie from each superfood group—fruit, veggies, whole grains, healthy fats, fish, and dairy—onto one plate to attack fat from all angles. Drop 10? With dishes like this, you can double that, easy.

2 tablespoons pumpkin seeds

$1/2$ cup cooked quinoa

$1/2$ cup grated Parmesan

$1/4$ cup oat flour

$1/2$ teaspoon garlic powder

1 egg

16 ounces wild salmon, skin removed, cut into 4 fillets

$1/4$ teaspoon salt

Vegetable oil cooking spray

1 tablespoon olive oil

4 cups broccoli florets (about 1 medium head)

$1/2$ cup uncooked whole-wheat couscous

$1/4$ cup goji berries

2 scallions (white and green parts), thinly sliced

2 teaspoons hot sauce

1 cup boiling water

Heat the oven to 425°F. Using a clean coffee grinder, grind the pumpkin seeds. Spread them out on a plate. Add the quinoa, Parmesan, flour, and garlic powder. Mix with your clean fingertips. In a separate, shallow dish, place the egg and whisk well.

Sprinkle the salmon with the salt and dredge one side of each piece in the egg. Press the egg-coated side into the pumpkin seed mixture.

Heat a large, oven-safe skillet over high heat. Remove from heat, coat with the cooking spray, and return to the stove. Add the salmon, coated-side down, and cook 2 to 3 minutes without disturbing. Carefully turn over the fish and slide the entire skillet into the oven. Bake 7 to 9 minutes, until the fish is still pink but no longer translucent in the center. Remove the pan from oven, take the fish out of the pan, and set aside.

Heat a second large skillet over high heat. Add the olive oil and the broccoli. Cook 2 to 3 minutes, stirring often, until the broccoli begins to brown. Reduce the heat to medium and add the couscous, goji berries, scallions, and hot sauce. Carefully add the boiling water and cover. Remove from the heat and allow to rest 10 minutes, until all the water is absorbed and the couscous is fluffy. Serve immediately with the salmon.

 464 CALORIES, 38 G PROTEIN, 19 G FAT (4 G SATURATED), 40 G CARBOHYDRATES, 7 G FIBER, 538 MG SODIUM

CHEF'S NOTE:
The goji-studded couscous makes a simple and satisfying
side for grilled chicken or shrimp, too.

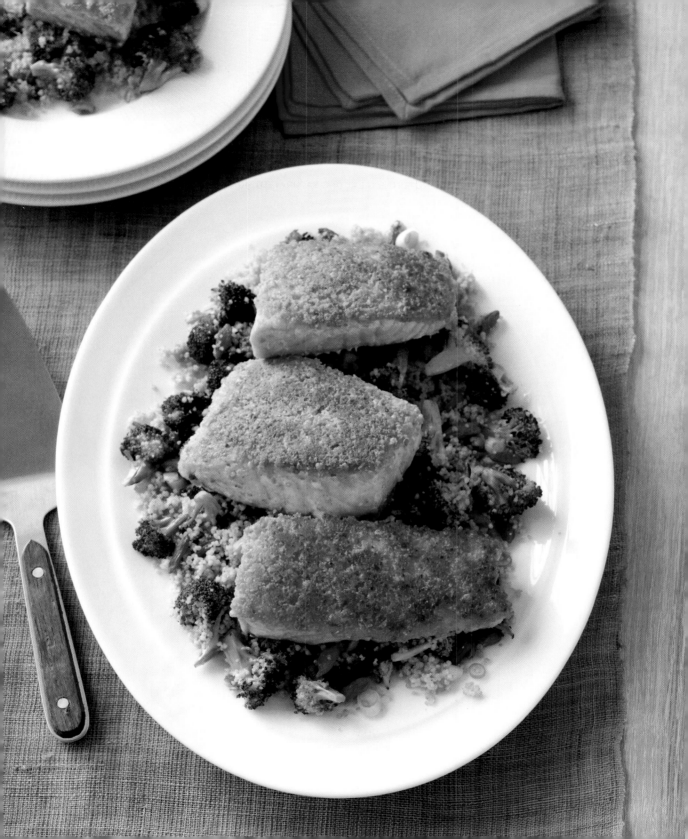

ROASTED LEMON CHICKEN WITH PEPPERCORN SWEET POTATOES

SERVES 4 • SUPERFOODS: Olive Oil, Sardines, Sweet Potatoes

Even if you're tempted to turn your nose up at sardines, give them a chance; it's easy to love the extra zest they bring to a simple chicken breast, and there's no denying the superstar status of their healthy omega-3s.

4 chicken breasts on the bone,
    skin removed
1 canned sardine, packed in water,
    drained
1 medium lemon, zested and juiced
    (about $1/4$ cup)
2 tablespoons fresh thyme leaves
    or tarragon leaves, chopped
2 cloves garlic, minced
3 medium sweet potatoes

2 tablespoons olive oil
1 tablespoon tomato
    paste
2 teaspoons black peppercorns,
    cracked with the back of a
    skillet
2 teaspoons paprika
1 teaspoon garlic powder
$1/2$ teaspoon cayenne
$1/4$ teaspoon salt

Heat the oven to 350°F. Place the chicken breasts on a baking sheet. In a small bowl, mash the sardine with the lemon zest and juice, thyme or tarragon, and garlic. Coat the top of each chicken breast with the mixture (using about 3 tablespoons per breast) and transfer it to the oven. Bake 40 to 45 minutes, until the chicken is cooked through and no longer pink inside.

    Scrub the potatoes under cold running water. Cut each potato into eight wedges and place them in a large bowl with the olive oil, tomato paste, cracked peppercorns, paprika, garlic powder, cayenne, and salt.

    Spread the wedges out on an ungreased baking sheet and bake 15 to 18 minutes, until the edges are brown and the potatoes are soft. Serve with the chicken.

 THE DISH 448 CALORIES, 43 G PROTEIN, 13 G FAT (2 G SATURATED), 40 G CARBOHYDRATES, 7 G FIBER, 556 MG SODIUM

CHEF'S NOTE:
Would you rather grill than roast? Use the topping as a marinade instead.

HARVEST CHICKEN WITH APPLE SWEET POTATO MASH

SERVES 4 • SUPERFOODS: Apples, Oats, Olive Oil, Pomegranate, Pumpkin Seeds, Sweet Potatoes

You'll never hear (or think), *Chicken again?* when you put this feast on the table. The sauce and mash add a sweet touch, while the protein in the bird and resistant starch in the spuds turn up the calorie-burning, fat-sizzling heat.

2 tablespoons extra-virgin olive oil, divided
1 red onion, cut into rings
1 apple, cored, chopped
2 medium sweet potatoes, peeled and chopped
$1/2$ cup water
4 boneless, skinless chicken breasts
$1/2$ teaspoon salt
$1/2$ cup oat flour
$1/4$ cup pumpkin seeds, chopped

THE SAUCE:
1 cup reduced-sodium chicken broth
$1/2$ cup balsamic vinegar
1 tablespoon cornstarch
$1/2$ cup pomegranate arils (from $1/4$ pomegranate)

Heat a large skillet over medium heat. Add half the olive oil, the onion, apple, and sweet potatoes. Reduce the heat to low and cook 4 to 6 minutes, stirring often, until the onion starts to brown. Add the water and cover. Simmer 10 to 15 minutes, until the sweet potatoes are tender. Transfer to a food processor and process until a thick mash forms. Set aside.

Heat the oven to 400°F. Sprinkle the chicken with the salt. Place the flour and pumpkin seeds on a shallow plate and mix together. Press both sides of the chicken into the flour mixture and transfer to a clean plate.

Heat a large, oven-safe skillet over high heat and add the remaining olive oil. Add the chicken breasts. Cook 4 to 6 minutes, turning once or twice, until a golden crust forms. Transfer to the oven and bake 5 to 6 minutes, until the chicken is cooked through and no longer pink in the center. Set out four plates and place one chicken breast on each. Return the skillet to the stove, with the heat off.

PREPARE THE SAUCE:

In a small bowl, whisk together the chicken broth, vinegar, and cornstarch until smooth. Add the broth to the skillet in which you cooked the chicken. Heat over medium heat and cook 1 to 2 minutes, stirring often, until the mixture thickens. Pour the sauce over the chicken breasts and sprinkle the pomegranate arils on top. Divide the sweet potato mash among the four plates and serve immediately.

 454 CALORIES, 41 G PROTEIN, 14 G FAT (2 G SATURATED), 44 G CARBOHYDRATES, 6 G FIBER, 725 MG SODIUM

ORANGE-GINGER CHICKEN WITH POMEGRANATE QUINOA

SERVES 4 • SUPERFOODS: Kale, Oats, Olive Oil, Pomegranate, Quinoa

You'll feel totally Zen about losing weight with this lean update on sweet-and-sour chicken. Kale balances the sweetness of the sauce, and protein-loaded quinoa is a flavorful, filling alternative to white rice.

$\frac{1}{2}$ cup uncooked white or red quinoa

1 $\frac{1}{4}$ cups water, divided

$\frac{1}{2}$ cup 100 percent pomegranate juice

2 oranges, zested and juiced (about 1 cup juice)

3 tablespoons light brown sugar

1 tablespoon cornstarch

2 tablespoons reduced-sodium soy sauce

2 garlic cloves, minced

1 teaspoon fresh gingerroot, minced

3 boneless, skinless chicken breasts (about 6 ounces each), cut into $\frac{1}{2}$-inch pieces

$\frac{1}{2}$ cup oat flour

2 tablespoons olive oil, divided

8 ounces kale (about 1 bunch), thinly sliced

2 scallions (white and green part), thinly sliced

Rinse the quinoa well under cold running water. In a 4-quart saucepan, bring 1 cup of the water to a boil and add the quinoa. Cover and cook 15 to 20 minutes, until the quinoa seeds are no longer opaque in the center. Stir in the pomegranate juice and set aside.

In a small bowl, place the orange zest and juice, brown sugar, cornstarch, soy sauce, garlic, and ginger. Add the remaining $\frac{1}{4}$ cup of water and mix. Set aside. Place the chicken on a plate and sprinkle it with the flour, turning the pieces to coat each well.

Heat a large skillet over high heat and add 1 tablespoon of oil and the kale. Cook 2 to 3 minutes, turning often, until the kale wilts. Transfer to a clean plate.

In the same skillet, add the remaining oil on medium-high heat. Add the flour-coated chicken and cook, 3 to 4 minutes, turning often, until the chicken browns. Reduce the heat to low and add the orange juice mixture. Cook 2 to 3 minutes, stirring often, until the chicken is cooked through and the sauce thickens. Divide the quinoa among four plates and top with the kale. Spoon a quarter of the cooked chicken on top. Garnish with the scallions. Serve immediately.

 457 CALORIES, 35 G PROTEIN, 13 G FAT (2 G SATURATED), 51 G CARBOHYDRATES, 6 G FIBER, 529 MG SODIUM

CHEF'S NOTE:
Red and white quinoa taste similar, but the red adds
appealing color to your plate.

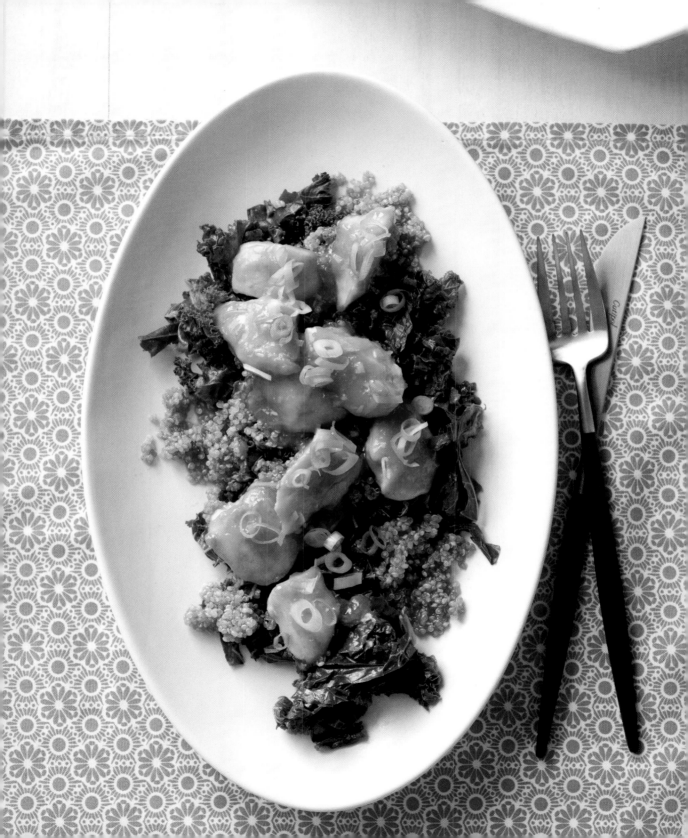

BUFFALO WILD SALMON FINGERS WITH AVOCADO SALAD

SERVES 4 • SUPERFOODS: Avocado, Eggs, Lentils, Oats,
Olive Oil, Wild Salmon, Yogurt

A cross between chicken fingers and fish sticks, this dish makes child's play out of eating nutritiously. The fiber (in lentils, avocados, and salmon) and healthy fats (in avocados and the fish) slow digestion, preventing a rush of blood sugar that packs fat on you.

> 6 cups mesclun greens
>
> 1 cup cooked red or brown lentils
>
> 1 ripe Hass avocado, cut into 1-inch cubes
>
> 2 6-ounce wild salmon fillets, skin removed
>
> 2 tablespoons hot sauce (for mild spiciness; use
> $^1/_4$ cup for hot)
>
> 1 egg
>
> 1 tablespoon plain, low-fat yogurt
>
> $^1/_4$ cup bread crumbs
>
> $^1/_2$ cup oat flour
>
> 2 tablespoons olive oil, divided

Place the greens, lentils, and avocado in a large bowl. Toss to combine. Divide the salad equally among four plates.

Cut each of the salmon fillets into six 4-inch-long strips. Place the hot sauce, egg, and yogurt in a shallow bowl. Whisk well. Place the bread crumbs and flour on a plate and mix with your fingertips.

Dip each fish strip into the egg mixture and then into the bread crumb mixture to coat. Transfer to a plate and repeat with remaining fish.

Heat a large skillet over medium heat and add half the oil and half the fish fingers. Cook 5 to 6 minutes, turning a few times, until the fish is cooked and flakes with a fork. Repeat with the remaining oil and fish. Transfer three fingers to each plate and serve.

449 CALORIES, 28 G PROTEIN, 25 G FAT (5 G SATURATED), 31 G CARBOHYDRATES, 8 G FIBER,
600 MG SODIUM

"SWEET" STEAK FRITES

SERVES 4 • SUPERFOODS: Kale, Mushrooms, Olive Oil, Steak, Sweet Potatoes

Each serving satisfies close to 100 percent of your fat-burning vitamin C quota, as well as supplying significant amounts of iron, zinc, and B vitamins.

1 cup dried mushrooms (1 ounce)

1 cup boiling water

4 center-cut filets mignons (about 4 ounces each)

½ teaspoon salt

1 tablespoon light olive oil

Nonstick cooking spray

1 large bunch kale, stems discarded, roughly chopped

8 ounces cremini or white button mushrooms, stems removed, quartered

16 ounces frozen sweet potato fries, cooked according to the package instructions (or see recipe, page 184)

Rinse the dried mushrooms well under cold running water. Place them in a bowl along with 1 cup boiling water. Set aside.

Heat the oven to 400°F. Sprinkle each filet with salt. Heat a large, oven-safe skillet over medium-high heat. Add the olive oil and the filets. Reduce the heat to medium and cook 2 to 3 minutes, without disturbing, until a golden crust forms. Flip the filets and cook until the meat begins to brown, 2 to 3 minutes. Slide the skillet into the oven and bake 5 to 6 minutes, until the meat is pink in the center but no longer red. Set out four plates and place one filet on each plate. Return the skillet to the stove, heat off.

Coat another large skillet with cooking spray and place it over high heat. Add the kale and cook 1 to 2 minutes, turning often, until the kale starts to wilt. Carefully add the liquid from the soaking mushrooms, reserving a few tablespoons, and cook 2 minutes, until the kale is soft and most of the liquid has evaporated. Set aside.

Coat the first skillet with cooking spray. Add the fresh mushrooms and cook 2 to 3 minutes, stirring often, until they soften. (If they stick, add the mushroom liquid.) Add the soaked mushrooms and toss well. Spoon the mushrooms over the filets. Divide the kale among the four plates and serve immediately with sweet potato fries.

449 CALORIES, 31 G PROTEIN, 17 G FAT (3 G SATURATED), 45 G CARBOHYDRATES, 7 G FIBER, 597 MG SODIUM

SAUSAGE AND BROCCOLI PASTA

SERVES 4 • SUPERFOODS: Broccoli, Olive Oil, Parmesan,
Sardines, Whole-Grain Pasta

Sausage, pasta, cheese—yep, these are diet foods! These surprise slimmers feel indulgent and come packed in a portion size big enough for the heartiest appetite.

8 ounces uncooked whole-wheat linguine or spaghetti

1 tablespoon olive oil

$1/2$ pound Italian turkey sausage (about 3 links)

1 teaspoon chili flakes

$1/2$ yellow or red onion, chopped

1 head broccoli, cut into florets, stem discarded

1 canned sardine, packed in oil

$1/3$ cup half-and-half

$1/2$ cup freshly grated Parmesan

Cook the pasta according to the package instructions. Reserve 1 cup of the cooking water before draining the pasta.

Heat a large skillet over medium heat. Add the olive oil. Add the sausage and cook 2 to 3 minutes, breaking it up with the back of a spoon. Sprinkle the chili flakes over the sausage and press them into the meat. Add the onion and cook 2 minutes, until it softens. Add the broccoli and sardine, and reduce the heat to low. Cook 2 minutes, stirring often, until the broccoli starts to soften.

Add the half-and-half to the skillet, and scrape up bits of sausage clinging to the bottom of the pan. Add the pasta and the Parmesan, and toss well. Add half of the reserved pasta water and toss again, adding a few tablespoons more if the mixture is dry. Divide the pasta among four plates or bowls and serve immediately.

452 CALORIES, 27 G PROTEIN, 17 G FAT (5 G SATURATED), 52 G CARBOHYDRATES, 7 G FIBER, 615 MG SODIUM

CHEF'S NOTE:

New to whole-grain pasta? Thinner noodles, such as linguine and spaghetti, are especially tender and taste more like traditional pasta than bulkier shapes like rotini.

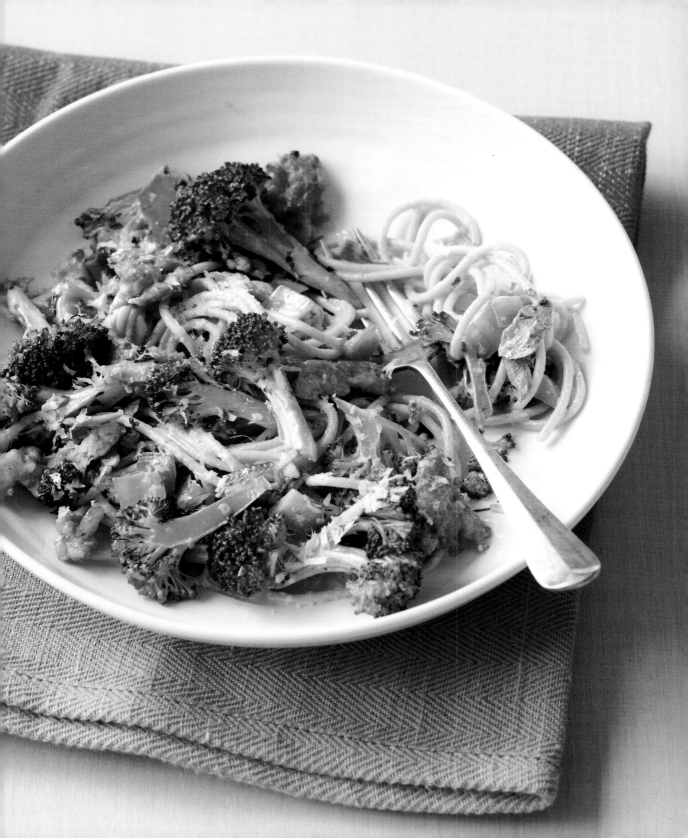

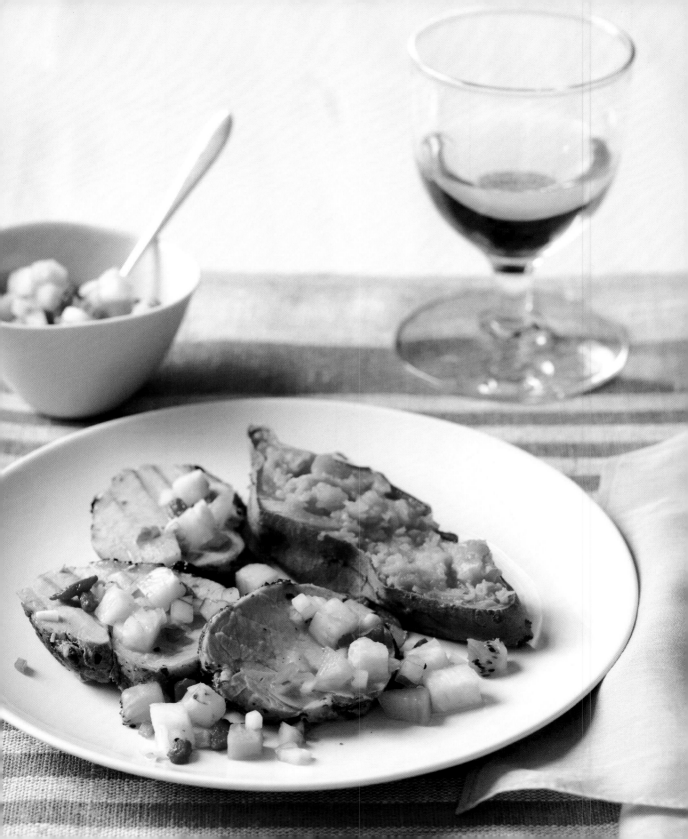

CILANTRO-GRILLED PORK LOIN WITH KIWI JALAPEÑO SALSA

SERVES 4 • SUPERFOODS: Goji Berries, Kiwifruit, Olive Oil, Sweet Potatoes

Every bite of the fruity relish nets you vitamin C, which will help you sizzle off extra fat the next time you work out. Plus, with a topping this sweet, you might not even want dessert. Maybe.

1 ½ pounds lean pork tenderloin

½ cup chopped cilantro

1 tablespoon light olive oil

2 garlic cloves, minced

½ teaspoon salt, divided

¼ teaspoon freshly ground black pepper

2 large sweet potatoes (about 20 ounces), cut in half lengthwise

2 kiwis, peeled, diced

2 cups pineapple cubes, diced

¼ cup (about 1 ounce) goji berries

½ small red onion, minced

1 jalapeño, minced

1 lime, zested and juiced

Heat the oven to 400˚F. In a shallow dish, place the pork, cilantro, olive oil, garlic, half the salt, and the black pepper. Rub the spices into the meat and cover. Refrigerate 2 hours.

Using a fork, poke a few holes in the sweet potatoes. Wrap each half in aluminum foil and bake 45 minutes to 1 hour, until the potatoes are soft to the touch. Remove the foil and set the potatoes aside to cool.

Prepare the salsa: Place the kiwis, pineapple, goji berries, onion, jalapeño, lime zest and juice, and remaining salt in a bowl. Stir to combine and set aside.

Heat a grill over high heat. Reduce the heat to medium and grill the pork 40 to 45 minutes, turning occasionally, until the meat is slightly pink but no longer translucent. Remove the pork from the grill and let rest 5 minutes before slicing. Using a fork, mash the sweet potatoes and return to the skins. Serve the pork with salsa and sweet potatoes.

 445 CALORIES, 39 G PROTEIN, 7 G FAT (2 G SATURATED), 56 G CARBOHYDRATES, 8 G FIBER, 811 MG SODIUM

CHEF'S NOTE:
Pork is a slim swap for chicken—it's leaner now than ever, and is inexpensive.

ROASTED WILD SALMON WITH BLUEBERRY-POMEGRANATE SAUCE

SERVES 4 • SUPERFOODS: Blueberries, Oats, Olive Oil, Pomegranate, Wild Salmon

The pretty, colorful sauce turns this dinner into an exotic experience. While you dig in, why not daydream of relaxing on an equally exotic beach? The fiber and antioxidants in the blueberries ensure excess fat won't tag along on any trip, real or imagined!

$^1/_2$ cup 100% pomegranate juice

$^1/_4$ cup balsamic vinegar

2 teaspoons cornstarch

4 cups baby spinach

2 tablespoons plus $^1/_2$ cup water

16 ounces wild salmon, skin on, cut into 4 pieces

$^1/_4$ teaspoon salt

$^1/_4$ cup oat flour

1 tablespoon olive oil

Nonstick cooking spray

2 garlic cloves, minced

2 teaspoons grated gingerroot

2 cups fresh or frozen (thawed) blueberries

6 ounces soba noodles, cooked according to package instructions

Place the pomegranate juice, balsamic vinegar, and the cornstarch in a small bowl and stir to combine. Set aside.

Heat the oven to 400°F. Heat a large, oven-safe skillet over medium-high heat. Add the spinach and 2 tablespoons of water. Cook 30 seconds, turning often, until the spinach wilts. Transfer to a plate.

Sprinkle the flesh side of the salmon with the salt and oat flour. Reheat the skillet on medium-high heat and add the olive oil. Add the salmon to the skillet, flesh-side down. Cook for 1 to 2 minutes, without turning, to allow a brown crust to form. Flip over the salmon and slide the skillet into the oven. Bake 6 to 8 minutes, until the salmon is pink but no longer translucent. Using a metal spatula, loosen the skin of the salmon to remove and discard it.

Reheat the skillet over medium heat. Remove from the heat, coat with cooking spray, and return to the stove. Add the garlic and ginger. Add the blueberries and $1/2$ cup of water. Cook 2 to 3 minutes, breaking up frozen blueberries (if used) with the back of a wooden spoon. Turn down the heat to low and stir in the pomegranate mixture. Cook 30 seconds, until a thick sauce forms. Divide the noodles among four plates and top each with $1/4$ cup wilted spinach and one salmon fillet. Finish each with $1/2$ cup of the sauce and serve immediately.

 459 CALORIES, 31 G PROTEIN, 12 G FAT (2 G SATURATED), 59 G CARBOHYDRATES, 6 G FIBER, 578 MG SODIUM

CHEF'S NOTE:
Fresh, in-season blueberries make this a perfect summer meal, but
for a culinary getaway any time of year, pick frozen berries.

PEANUT CHICKEN FINGERS

SERVES 4 • SUPERFOODS: Broccoli, Eggs, Olive Oil, Peanuts

Craving the crunch of fried food, but not the fat? The peanut-and-bread-crumb coating on this filling finger food is every bit as appealing as typical chicken strips, but extra low in calories.

 2 slices whole-grain bread
 $1/2$ cup peanuts
 2 garlic cloves
 3 boneless, skinless chicken breasts (about 6 ounces each)
 $1/8$ teaspoon salt
 2 eggs
 2 tablespoons water
 Nonstick cooking spray
 4 teaspoons olive oil
 1 head broccoli, florets only, steamed

Place the bread, peanuts, and garlic in a food processor and pulse fifteen to twenty times, until coarse bread crumbs form.

Cut the chicken into twelve 4-inch-long strips and sprinkle with the salt. Place the eggs in a shallow bowl with 2 tablespoons of water and whisk. Dip the chicken strips one at a time into the egg, then press into the bread crumbs. Transfer to a plate and chill at least 30 minutes to help the bread crumbs adhere to the chicken.

Heat two large skillets over high heat. Remove each from the heat, coat with cooking spray, and return to the stove. Add 2 teaspoons of oil to each. Divide the breaded strips between the two skillets and cook 3 to 4 minutes, without disturbing, until the bread crumbs crisp. Flip over and cook 3 to 4 minutes, until the chicken is cooked through and no longer translucent in the center. Transfer the chicken to a serving platter and sprinkle with salt. Serve with broccoli.

390 CALORIES, 36 G PROTEIN, 19 G FAT (3 G SATURATED), 20 G CARBOHYDRATES, 5 G FIBER, 359 MG SODIUM

SAGE CHICKEN WITH LENTILS AND PROSCIUTTO

SERVES 4 • SUPERFOODS: Artichokes, Cherries, Lentils, Olive Oil

Inspired by chicken saltimbocca, the classic prosciutto-stuffed Italian favorite, this dish teams up fiber-rich artichokes, cherries, and lentils to help inspire you to meet your pounds-off goals.

4 boneless, skinless chicken
    breasts (about 6 ounces each)
4 sage leaves
4 garlic cloves, thinly sliced
4 teaspoons olive oil, divided
½ red onion, chopped
½ cup dry lentils, rinsed well under
    cold running water

1 cup water
1 9-ounce package frozen
    artichoke hearts,
    thawed
2 ounces prosciutto, excess fat
    removed, chopped
2 teaspoons Dijon mustard
½ cup dried cherries

Make a deep, horizontal slice into the side of each chicken breast. Press a sage leaf and a few slices of garlic into each. Wrap each chicken breast in plastic and pound to seal the edges.

Heat a large skillet over high heat and add half the olive oil. Add the chicken and cook, turning occasionally, until the chicken browns and is no longer translucent in the center, 7 to 8 minutes.

Heat another large skillet over medium-high heat. Add the remaining olive oil and onion. Cook 4 to 6 minutes, stirring often, until the onion is soft. Add the lentils and water. Cover and cook 15 to 20 minutes, until the lentils are tender and the water has been absorbed. Add the artichokes, prosciutto, mustard, and dried cherries and stir well. Cook 1 minute, until the artichokes are warm.

Set out four plates and place one chicken breast on each. Divide the lentil mixture among the plates and serve immediately.

THE DISH
461 CALORIES, 48 G PROTEIN, 12 G FAT (2 G SATURATED), 38 G CARBOHYDRATES, 12 G FIBER, 676 MG SODIUM

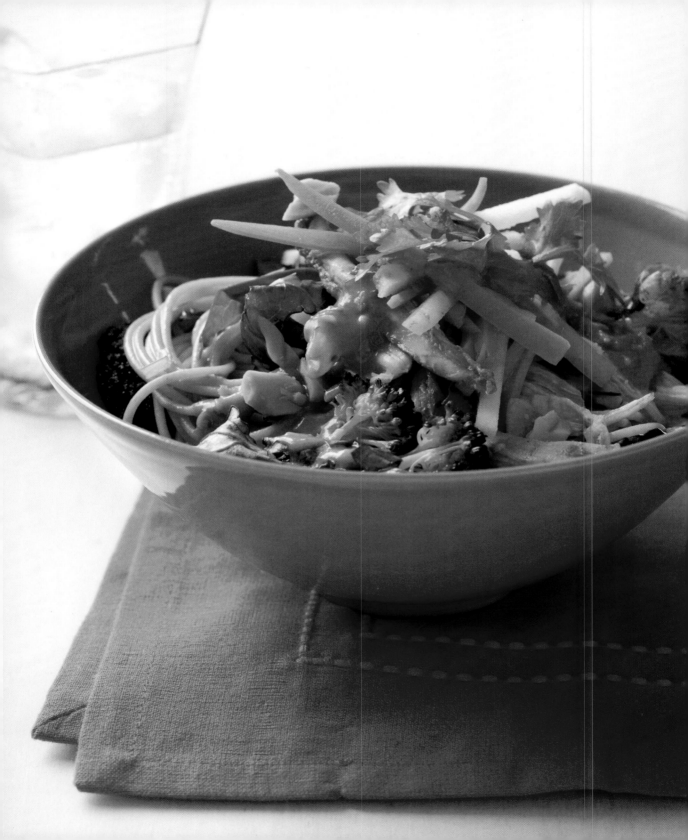

THAI CHICKEN SALAD

SERVES 4 • SUPERFOODS: Apples, Broccoli, Kale, Olive Oil, Peanuts, Whole-Grain Pasta

This salad may be full of hunger-taming veggies, but thanks to the rich peanut dressing, each forkful feels more decadent than diet-y. Tart and crunchy Granny Smith apples add a cool zing to counter the spice from the chili paste.

2 boneless, skinless, chicken breasts

6 teaspoons hot chili paste, such as sambal (or Sriracha), divided

Vegetable oil cooking spray

2 tablespoons light olive oil, divided

2 cups broccoli florets, chopped

2 cups kale, chopped

4 ounces dry thin, whole-wheat spaghetti, cooked according to package instructions

2 limes, zested and juiced (about 1/2 cup)

2 tablespoons reduced-sodium soy sauce

2 tablespoons smooth peanut butter

2 garlic cloves, minced

1 teaspoon sugar

4 carrots, peeled and cut into matchsticks

1 Granny Smith apple, shredded or cut into matchsticks

1/2 cup packed cilantro leaves

1/4 cup coarsely chopped roasted, unsalted peanuts

Heat the oven to 400°F. Coat the chicken with half of the chili paste. Heat a medium, oven-safe skillet over high heat. Remove from the heat and coat with cooking spray. Return to the heat and add the chicken. Cook 3 to 4 minutes, turning once, to brown both sides.

Place the skillet in the oven and bake about 6 minutes, until the chicken is cooked through and no longer pink. Remove the skillet from the oven and rest the chicken on a cutting board for 5 minutes. Shred and set aside.

Reheat the skillet over medium-high heat. Add 1 tablespoon of the olive oil. Add the broccoli and kale and reduce the heat to low. Cover and cook 3 to 4 minutes, stirring often, until the broccoli and kale are soft. Add the pasta. Remove from the heat and keep covered.

Prepare the dressing: In a small bowl, whisk the remaining chili paste, olive oil, lime zest and juice, soy sauce, peanut butter, garlic, and sugar until smooth.

Divide the pasta and vegetables among four plates. Add a quarter of the carrots and shredded chicken to each plate. Top with the apple, cilantro, and peanuts. Drizzle with the dressing. Serve immediately.

 347 CALORIES, 30 G PROTEIN, 19 G FAT (3 G SATURATED), 46 G CARBOHYDRATES, 8 G FIBER, 657 MG SODIUM

PAN-ROASTED SHIITAKE CHICKEN WITH APPLE-CELERY ROOT PUREE

SERVES 4 • SUPERFOODS: Apples, Broccoli, Mushrooms, Olive Oil, Parmesan

If you still bake the chicken casserole with cream of mushroom soup your mother used to make, you're due for an upgrade. Even Mom will love how the dense, rich shiitake mushrooms fill you up for a scant 78 calories per chopped cup.

Olive oil cooking spray

2 celery roots, each about the size of a small grapefruit, peeled, diced

1 tablespoon brown sugar

$1/2$ cup water

2 apples, cored, diced

$1/4$ cup grated Parmesan

4 skinless, boneless chicken breasts

$1/4$ teaspoon salt

1 tablespoon olive oil

2 garlic cloves, minced

3 cups (8 ounces) shiitake mushrooms, stems discarded, caps finely chopped

$1/2$ cup half-and-half

1 head broccoli, florets only, steamed

Coat a large skillet with cooking spray and place over medium heat. Add the celery roots and brown sugar and cook 3 to 4 minutes, stirring often, until the celery roots start to brown. Carefully add $1/2$ cup of water and cover. Cook 4 to 5 minutes, until the celery roots are fork-tender and most of the liquid has evaporated. Remove the lid and add the apples. Cook 2 minutes, stirring often, until the apple softens. Transfer to the bowl of a food processor and add the Parmesan. Blend until a mash forms and set aside.

Sprinkle the chicken with the salt. Heat another large skillet over medium heat. Remove from the heat, coat with cooking spray, and return to the stove. Add the chicken and cook 3 to 4 minutes, turning once or twice, until the chicken starts to brown. Transfer the chicken to a plate. In the same skillet, add the olive oil and garlic. Add the mushrooms and cook 2 to 3 minutes, until the mushrooms soften. Add the half-and-half and turn off the heat.

Return the chicken to the skillet and cook 5 to 6 minutes, until the chicken is cooked through and no longer pink inside, and the sauce thickens. Serve immediately with the broccoli and apple-celery root puree.

 464 CALORIES, 46 G PROTEIN, 14 G FAT (5 G SATURATED), 42 G CARBOHYDRATES, 9 G FIBER, 639 MG SODIUM

GARLICKY FLANK STEAK WITH SWEET POTATO, ORANGE, AND LENTIL SALAD

SERVES 4 • SUPERFOODS: Edamame, Lentils, Olive Oil, Steak, Sweet Potatoes

Sweet potatoes and oranges are a match made in health heaven! Both contain vitamin C, which helps your body better absorb beef's energizing iron. Vitamin C also helps you get extra toned by feeding your furnace more fat while you exercise.

1 pound flank steak

4 garlic cloves, minced

1/2 cup parsley, chopped

4 teaspoons olive oil, divided

1 teaspoon Dijon mustard

1/2 teaspoon salt, divided

1 large sweet potato (about 10 ounces), peeled, cut into 1/2-inch cubes

1/2 cup dry lentils

2 cups water

1 cup frozen, shelled edamame, defrosted

2 tablespoons orange marmalade

2 oranges, cut into segments

Place the steak, garlic, parsley, 2 teaspoons olive oil, and mustard in a zipper-lock bag. Shake the bag to evenly coat the steak. Marinate, refrigerated, overnight.

Heat the oven to 400°F. Remove the steak from the bag and scrape off any garlic. Reserve the garlic and marinade. Sprinkle the steak with half the salt.

Heat a large, oven-safe skillet over medium-high heat. Add the steak and brown 2 minutes per side. Turn off the heat and top the steak with the reserved garlic and marinade. Transfer the skillet with the steak into the oven. Bake 10 to 12 minutes, until the steak is pink but no longer translucent inside. Allow to rest 5 minutes on a cutting board before slicing.

Heat a large skillet over medium-high heat. Add the remaining olive oil and the sweet potato. Brown the sweet potato for about 1 minute, stirring occasionally. Add the lentils and water. Reduce the heat to low and cover. Simmer 20 minutes, until the sweet potato and lentils are soft but still hold their shape. Stir in the remaining salt, the edamame, marmalade, and orange segments. Divide among four plates. Distribute the sliced steak to each plate and serve immediately.

THE DISH

474 CALORIES, 37 G PROTEIN, 16 G FAT (5 G SATURATED), 47 G CARBOHYDRATES, 12 G FIBER, 429 MG SODIUM

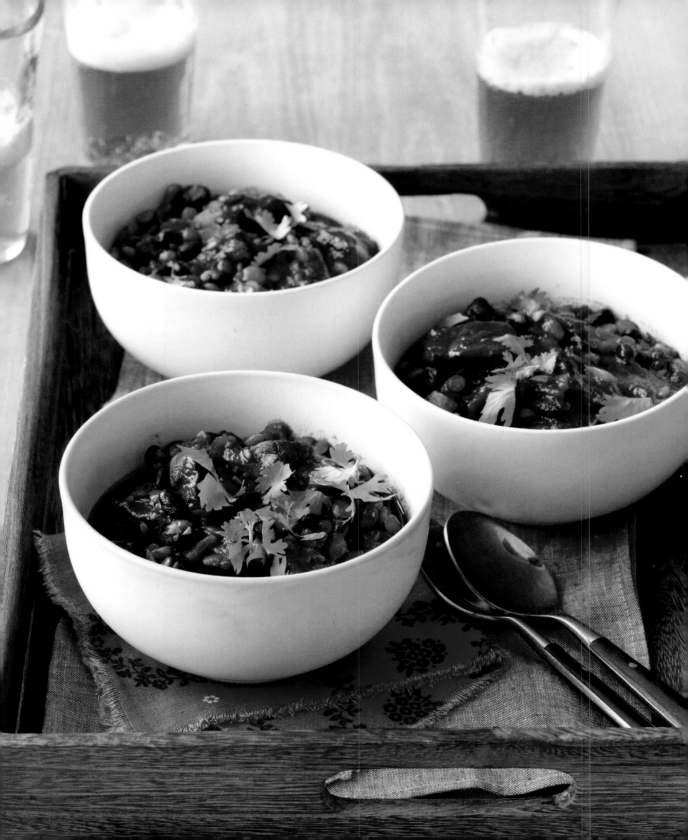

CHUNKY BEEF CHILI

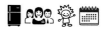

SERVES 4 • SUPERFOODS: Coffee, Lentils, Olive Oil, Steak

You're probably thinking, *Coffee? In chili?* Try it: The brew brings out the flavor of beef. The black beans and lentils add even more calorie-melting power, securing this meaty bowl a spot in the protein hall of fame.

1 pound lean beef stew meat, trimmed of excess fat, cut into 1-inch cubes

¼ teaspoon salt

1 teaspoon paprika

¼ teaspoon freshly ground black pepper

1 tablespoon olive oil

1 medium yellow or red onion, chopped

3 garlic cloves, chopped

1 teaspoon chopped fresh oregano

1 chipotle chile en adobo

1 tablespoon tomato paste

1 tablespoon brown sugar

¼ cup brewed coffee

1 15-ounce can diced tomatoes

¾ cup uncooked red or brown lentils

2 ½ cups water

1 15-ounce can reduced-sodium black beans

Cilantro leaves

Sprinkle the beef with the salt, paprika, and black pepper.

Heat a stockpot over medium-high heat and add the olive oil. Add the beef and cook 4 to 5 minutes, turning once or twice, until it is well browned. Transfer the beef to a plate.

Reduce the heat to medium. Add the onion, garlic, and oregano to the saucepan and cook 2 to 3 minutes, stirring often, until the onion starts to soften.

Return the meat to the stockpot, along with any juices that accumulated on the plate. Add the chipotle chile and tomato paste and cook 1 minute, stirring often. Add the brown sugar, coffee, and diced tomatoes (with juice). Cover and reduce the heat to low. Simmer about 30 minutes, until the liquid has reduced by half.

Add the lentils and water and simmer, covered, 30 minutes, stirring occasionally. Add the beans and cook 1 minute. Garnish with cilantro, if desired, and serve.

THE DISH   450 CALORIES, 40 G PROTEIN, 10 G FAT (2 G SATURATED), 51 G CARBOHYDRATES, 19 G FIBER, 706 MG SODIUM

TANGY TURKEY MEAT LOAF

SERVES 4 • SUPERFOODS: Eggs, Lentils, Mushrooms, Oats

You won't taste the mushrooms and lentils in this twist on the diner classic, but they'll work their fat-melting magic anyway. The lentils boost your calorie burn, while the satiating mushrooms help keep the turkey moist.

> 1 pound 93% lean ground turkey
> 1 cup old-fashioned oats
> 1 cup cooked red lentils
> 3 ounces cremini or button mushrooms, finely chopped
>   (1 $^1/_4$ cups)
> 2 garlic cloves, minced
> 1 egg
> 1 teaspoon chopped fresh rosemary or thyme
> $^1/_4$ teaspoon ground cayenne
> $^1/_2$ cup barbecue sauce or ketchup, divided
> Nonstick cooking spray

Heat the oven to 350°F. Place the turkey, oats, lentils, mushrooms, garlic, egg, rosemary (or thyme), cayenne, and half the barbecue sauce in a large bowl. Mix well with your hands until the mixture is smooth and even.

Coat a 1-pound loaf pan with cooking spray. Add the turkey mixture and form into a loaf. Using a rubber spatula, spread the remaining barbecue sauce over top. Bake about 45 minutes, until the meat loaf starts to pull away from the sides and is firm to the touch. Rest 5 minutes before slicing and serve immediately.

THE DISH

306 CALORIES, 28 G PROTEIN, 9 G FAT (2 G SATURATED), 29 G CARBOHYDRATES, 4 G FIBER, 567 MG SODIUM

CHEF'S NOTE:
Ninety-three percent lean ground turkey is a standard supermarket offering, but if you can find one with even less fat, go for it!

LEMONY SOLE WITH CAPERS, ARTICHOKES, AND SWEET POTATOES

SERVES 4 • SUPERFOODS: Artichokes, Oats, Olive Oil, Parmesan, Sweet Potatoes

This fresh catch in a rich, creamy sauce looks and tastes like the special at a fancy fish house, but it cooks up quickly at home. If you're not familiar with sole, use this recipe to get to know the delicately flavored seafood, which weighs in at less than 100 calories per 4-ounce fillet.

16 ounces of fillet of sole, cut into 4 pieces

1/3 cup oat flour

2 tablespoons olive oil

1 9-ounce package frozen artichoke hearts, defrosted, chopped

2 tablespoons capers, rinsed well under cold running water, chopped

1 lemon, zested and juiced

1/3 cup half-and-half

1/4 cup parsley, chopped

POTATOES:

2 large sweet potatoes, peeled, sliced into wedges

Nonstick cooking spray

1 cup grated Parmesan

1/4 teaspoon salt

Sprinkle the fillets with flour, coating both sides.

Heat a large skillet over medium-high heat. Add the oil and fish and cook 4 to 6 minutes, turning once or twice, until both sides are browned. (When done, the fish will easily flake when poked with a fork.) Remove the fish from the skillet and place on a plate.

Reduce heat to low. In the same skillet, place the artichokes, capers, and lemon zest and juice and cook 1 minute, until volume reduces by one-half. Turn off the heat and slowly whisk in the half-and-half. Spoon over fish and garnish with parsley.

PREPARE POTATOES:

Heat the oven to 400°F. Place the potato wedges on a baking sheet and coat with cooking spray. Bake for 45 minutes to 1 hour, until the potatoes are soft to the touch. Remove from the oven and let cool 10 minutes. Sprinkle with the Parmesan and the salt. Serve immediately with the fish.

 457 CALORIES, 35 G PROTEIN, 17 G FAT (6 G SATURATED), 42 G CARBOHYDRATES, 10 G FIBER, 796 MG SODIUM

CHEF'S NOTE:
Short on time? Substitute frozen sweet potato fries.

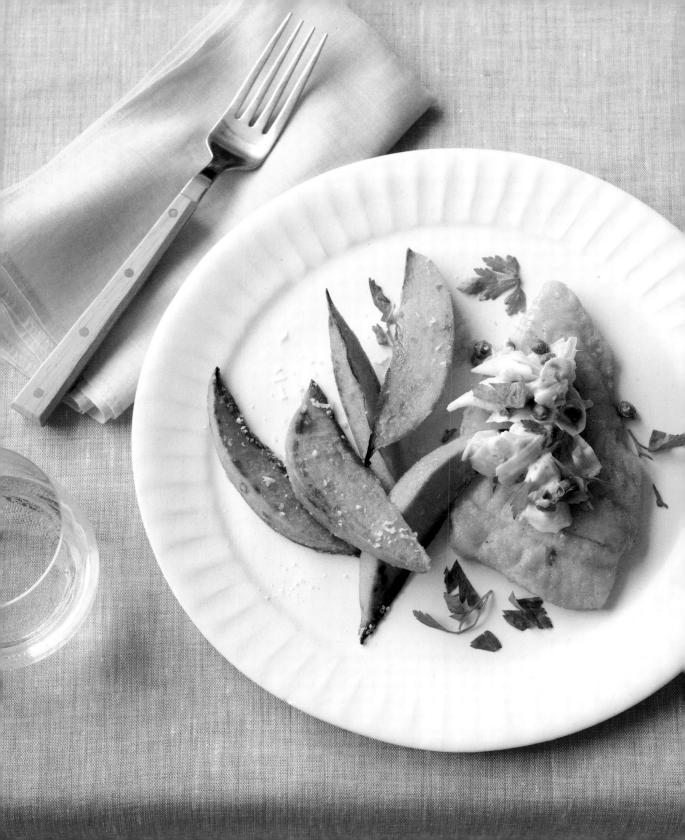

MUSHROOM-TURKEY MEATBALLS WITH ANGEL-HAIR PASTA

SERVES 6 (makes 18 meatballs) • SUPERFOODS: Eggs, Mushrooms, Oats, Olive Oil, Parmesan, Whole-Grain Pasta

This light, filling dish contains plenty of fiber, plus calcium to trigger fat burning.

1/2 cup old-fashioned oats

1/2 cup grated Parmesan, divided

1 egg

2 garlic cloves, minced

1/4 teaspoon salt

1 pound 93% lean ground turkey

8 ounces cremini or white button mushrooms, caps and stems, finely chopped (2 3/4 cups)

2 cups baby spinach, finely chopped

2 tablespoons extra-virgin olive oil, divided

1 28-ounce can diced tomatoes

1/2 cup water

1 sprig basil

10 ounces whole-wheat angel-hair pasta, cooked according to the package instructions

Place the oats, half the Parmesan, the egg, garlic, and salt in a large bowl. Mix well to coat the oats with the egg. Add the turkey, mushrooms, and spinach. Mix well with your hands until the mixture is smooth and the oats and mushrooms are evenly distributed.

Roll the mixture into balls the size of a golf balls. Heat a stockpot over medium-high heat and add 1 tablespoon of the oil. Add half the meatballs and cook 1 minute without disturbing. Cook 2 to 3 minutes, turning occasionally, until they are browned. Transfer to a clean plate and repeat with the remaining oil and when the second batch is browned, add back the first cooked batch. Carefully add the canned tomatoes with their juices and the water. Add the basil. Reduce the heat to medium and bring to a steady simmer.

Reduce the heat to medium-low and simmer, covered, 20 to 25 minutes until the meatballs are cooked through and the sauce thickens. Discard the basil and transfer the meatballs to a bowl. Toss the pasta in the remaining sauce and serve with meatballs.

441 CALORIES, 28 G PROTEIN, 16 G FAT (5 G SATURATED), 48 G CARBOHYDRATES, 7 G FIBER, 620 MG SODIUM

CRISPY POPCORN SHRIMP WITH NOODLES

SERVES 4 • SUPERFOODS: Eggs, Olive Oil, Popcorn, Whole-Grain Pasta

And the award for the most creative use of a superfood goes to . . . this delicious reinvention of greasy popcorn shrimp. Ground up with spices, popcorn transforms into a healthy, whole-grain breading that adds crunch and fiber to the low-calorie seafood.

4 cups popped popcorn
1/2 cup packed cilantro leaves
1 tablespoon fresh rosemary
1 teaspoon garlic powder
1 egg
1 pound large raw shrimp (about 16), tails on
3 tablespoons olive oil, divided
2 carrots, peeled, thinly sliced or shredded

1 red bell pepper, thinly sliced or shredded
1 small red onion, diced
4 cups baby spinach
2 tablespoons water
3 tablespoons barbecue sauce
6 ounces dry whole-wheat spaghetti, cooked according to the package instructions

Place the popcorn, cilantro, rosemary, and garlic powder in a food processor. Process 20 to 30 seconds, until the popcorn is finely chopped. Transfer to a plate.

Place the egg in a shallow dish and whisk well. Dip the shrimp into the egg, and then into the popcorn mixture. Transfer to a plate and refrigerate, uncovered, at least 30 minutes.

Heat a large skillet over high heat. Add half the olive oil and the shrimp. Reduce the heat to medium and cook, turning occasionally, until the shrimp is cooked through, 5 to 7 minutes. Transfer to a plate.

Heat a second large skillet over high heat. Add the remaining olive oil and the carrots, bell pepper, and onion. Reduce the heat to medium and cook 4 to 6 minutes, stirring the vegetables often, until they soften. Add the spinach and water. Cook 30 seconds, stirring often, until the spinach wilts. Add the barbecue sauce and pasta and toss to coat. Toss or plate with shrimp and serve.

THE DISH

450 CALORIES, 27 G PROTEIN, 14 G FAT (2 G SATURATED), 57 G CARBOHYDRATES, 9 G FIBER, 852 MG SODIUM

PISTACHIO- AND PUMPKIN-SEED-CRUSTED LAMB CHOP WITH CHERRY QUINOA

SERVES 4 • SUPERFOODS: Cherries, Eggs, Oats, Pumpkin Seeds, Quinoa

Think of this recipe as the paint-by-numbers of cooking: simple to execute, pretty and praiseworthy when complete. The gourmet nut-and-seed crust adds protein, fiber, and heart-helping fats; pistachio's oleic acid may also help you stay fuller after you eat.

2 tablespoons shelled, unsalted pistachio nuts
2 tablespoons pumpkin seeds
2 garlic cloves
2 tablespoons oat flour
1 egg
1 rack of lamb (1 $^3/_4$ pounds, 8 chops), trimmed of fat
Olive oil cooking spray
$^1/_2$ teaspoon salt, divided

6 cups baby spinach
2 tablespoons water
$^1/_2$ cup dry quinoa, rinsed well under cold running water, cooked according to the package instructions
$^1/_4$ cup dried cherries
4 scallions, white and green parts, thinly sliced
$^1/_4$ cup fresh mint leaves, chopped

Heat the oven to 375°F. Sprinkle half the salt on the lamb.

Place the pistachios, pumpkin seeds, and garlic in a food processor. Pulse until a crumbly mixture forms. Add the flour and pulse again. Spread onto a sheet of waxed paper.

Place the egg on a shallow plate and whisk well. Dip the lamb into the egg and press into the nut mixture. Transfer the lamb to a baking sheet with sides and coat the lamb with cooking spray. Sprinkle the lamb with half the salt. Bake 40 to 45 minutes, until the meat is pink but no longer red in the center. Rest the lamb for 10 minutes. Cut into chops and place two chops on each of four plates.

Heat a skillet over high heat. Add the spinach and 2 tablespoons of water. Cook 20 to 30 seconds, turning often, until the spinach wilts.

Stir together the spinach, quinoa, cherries, scallions, and remaining salt. Garnish with the mint leaves. Serve immediately with the lamb and spinach.

 462 CALORIES, 54 G PROTEIN, 15 G FAT (5 G SATURATED), 30 G CARBOHYDRATES, 5 G FIBER, 554 MG SODIUM

WILD SALMON AND PAN-ROASTED BRUSSELS SPROUTS WITH GOJIS

SERVES 4 • SUPERFOODS: Cherries, Goji Berries, Olive Oil, Pomegranate, Quinoa, Wild Salmon

Brussels sprouts, like other members of the cruciferous cabbage family, bolster your body's defenses against cancer. The omega-3s in wild salmon and the vitamin C in the sweet glaze also enhance your health while helping protect you from weight creep.

1 cup dry quinoa (about 3 cups cooked)
1/4 cup 100% pomegranate juice
1/4 cup water
1/4 cup goji berries
1/2 cup dark cherries, chopped
2 tablespoons honey

2 tablespoons low-sodium soy sauce
16 ounces wild salmon
Nonstick cooking spray
2 teaspoons olive oil
2 pints brussels sprouts, trimmed, quartered

Rinse the quinoa well under cold running water. Cook according to the package instructions. Stir in the pomegranate juice and set aside.

In a small saucepan, bring the water to a boil. Turn off the heat. Add the goji berries and cherries and allow to rest 10 minutes, until the berries plump up. Transfer the berries and cherries, with their liquid, to a blender. Add the honey and soy sauce and blend until a chunky sauce forms.

Heat the oven to 400°F. Place the salmon in an 8 × 11-inch baking dish. Coat the top with cooking spray and bake 6 to 8 minutes, until the fish is pink and no longer translucent in the center. During the last 2 minutes, drizzle on the goji berry sauce.

While the salmon cooks, heat a large skillet over medium heat. Add the olive oil and the brussels sprouts and cook 5 to 6 minutes, until the brussels sprouts start to brown. Reduce the heat to low and add the quinoa. Toss to combine.

Divide the fish and the vegetable-quinoa mixture among four plates and serve immediately.

THE DISH

461 CALORIES, 34 G PROTEIN, 12 G FAT (2 G SATURATED), 55 G CARBOHYDRATES, 7 G FIBER, 374 MG SODIUM

VEGETABLE LO MEIN

SERVES 4 • SUPERFOODS: Broccoli, Mushrooms,
Olive Oil, Whole-Grain Pasta

Your dream dinner order—flavorful, carb-tastic lo mein, hold the grease—is coming right up! Oyster sauce and light olive oil are satisfyingly rich and creamy, without adding a lot of calories or saturated fat, and the veggies are super filling.

1/4 cup light olive oil

1 head broccoli, cut into florets, stem discarded

1/2 pound shiitake mushrooms, stems discarded, caps
    thinly sliced

4 carrots, peeled and shredded

1 red bell pepper, seeded, thinly sliced

4 cups packed baby spinach

4 scallions (green and white parts), thinly sliced

2 garlic cloves, minced

1 1-inch piece gingerroot, minced

8 ounces thin dry whole-wheat fettuccine, cooked
    according to the package instructions

3 tablespoons oyster sauce

2 tablespoons reduced-sodium soy sauce

1/2 cup water

Heat a large skillet over high heat. Add the olive oil, broccoli, mushrooms, carrots, and bell pepper. Cook 2 to 3 minutes, stirring often, until the vegetables start to soften. Add the spinach and cook 1 minute, stirring often, until the spinach wilts. Add the scallions, garlic, and ginger. Cook about 1 minute, until fragrant. Add the pasta and reduce the heat to low. Add the oyster sauce, soy sauce, and water. Toss and serve immediately.

 THE DISH 466 CALORIES, 17 G PROTEIN, 15 G FAT (2 G SATURATED), 73 G CARBOHYDRATES, 14 G FIBER, 780 MG SODIUM

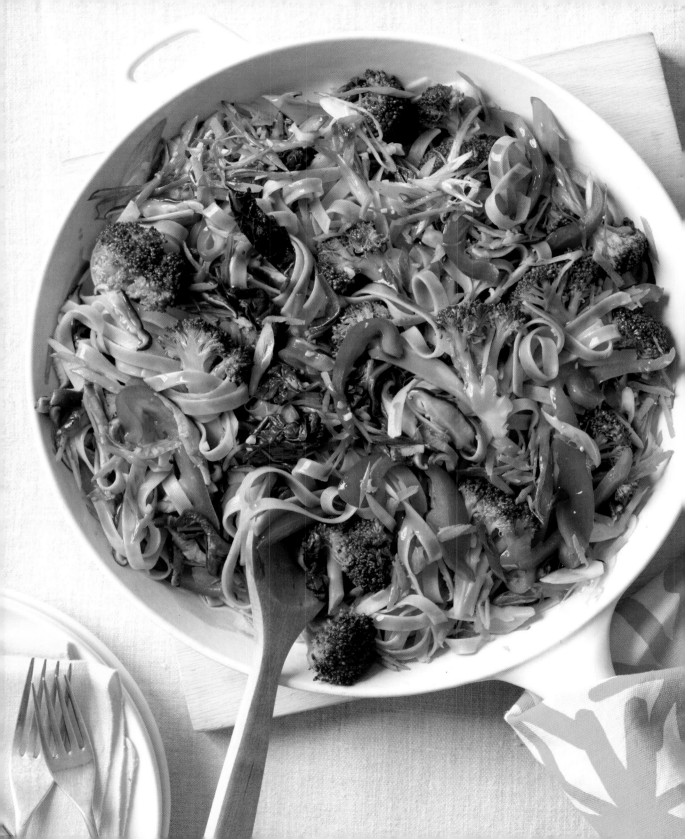

WILD SALMON CEVICHE WITH MANGO AND AVOCADO

SERVES 4 • SUPERFOODS: Avocado, Goji Berries, Peanuts, Wild Salmon

Fresh and tangy, ceviche is an easy, get-lean lunch that is practically impossible to screw up. This one adds peanuts to the traditional mix, lending a toasty crunch as well as fiber and healthy fats to help you resist cravings.

8 ounces sushi-grade wild salmon

2 large, ripe mangoes, peeled and cubed

$^1\!/_4$ red onion, thinly sliced

$^1\!/_4$ cup goji berries

$^1\!/_4$ cup chopped peanuts

2 tablespoons finely minced cilantro

1 lime, zested and juiced

$^1\!/_4$ teaspoon salt

1 ripe Hass avocado, peeled and cubed

4 ounces multigrain pita chips

Cut the salmon into $^1\!/_2$-inch cubes and place in a large bowl. Add the mangoes, onion, goji berries, peanuts, cilantro, lime zest and juice, and salt. Toss to coat. Refrigerate at least 1 hour. Before serving, gently fold in the avocado. Plate with the pita chips.

THE DISH

450 CALORIES, 19 G PROTEIN, 22 G FAT (3 G SATURATED), 47 G CARBOHYDRATES, 7 G FIBER, 466 MG SODIUM

CHEF'S NOTE:

Sushi-grade salmon has been pre-frozen to kill any parasites. If your fishmonger doesn't carry it, place an order for salmon sashimi with a local sushi restaurant.

POACHED GREEN TEA WILD SALMON WITH CUCUMBERS AND KIWI

SERVES 4 • SUPERFOODS: Almond Butter, Kiwifruit, Wild Salmon

Steeped in tea, this recipe's noodles and pretty salmon take on its subtle flavor. The cucumber-and-kiwi topping balances the rich, almond-butter-based sauce, which contains alpha-linolenic acid, a nutrient that may speed the metabolism of fats.

    4 quarts water

    4 green tea bags

    6 ounces uncooked soba noodles

    4 fillets wild salmon, skin on (4 ounces each)

    1 lime, zested and juiced

    3 tablespoons almond butter

    2 tablespoons reduced-sodium soy sauce

    1 large cucumber, peeled and cubed

    2 kiwis, peeled and thinly sliced

    2 scallions (green and white parts), thinly sliced

In a large stockpot, bring 4 quarts of water to a boil. Add the tea bags and steep 5 minutes. Remove the tea bags and bring the tea back to a boil. Add the noodles and cook 4 to 5 minutes, until the noodles are soft.

Add the salmon and turn the heat off. Cover and rest 20 minutes, until the salmon is cooked through. Remove the salmon and set aside.

In a large bowl, place the lime zest and juice, almond butter, and soy sauce. Whisk well to combine. Remove the noodles from the green tea and add them to the bowl. Add ¼ cup of the green tea. Gently toss to combine. Divide the noodles among four bowls. Top each with a salmon fillet, the cucumber, kiwis, and scallions. Serve immediately.

THE DISH

444 CALORIES, 33 G PROTEIN, 15 G FAT (2 G SATURATED), 48 G CARBOHYDRATES, 5 G FIBER, 257 MG SODIUM

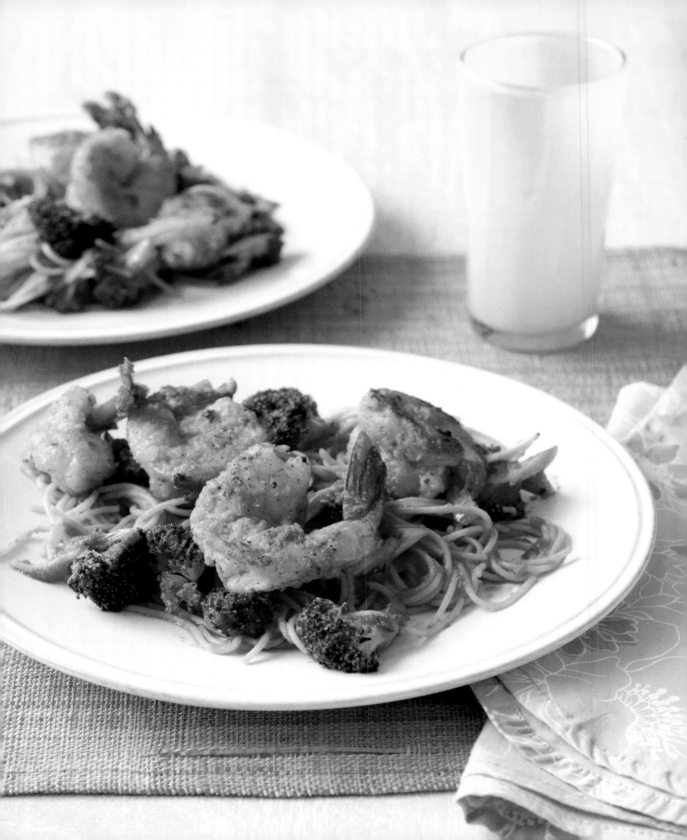

SHRIMP PARMESAN WITH BROCCOLI

SERVES 4 • SUPERFOODS: Broccoli, Eggs, Oats,
Olive Oil, Parmesan, Whole-Grain Pasta

Love chicken parm? This feast plates up the same flavors, but makes a few lean swaps. The shrimp's healthy fats help your body burn fat more efficiently, and the whole-wheat noodles deliver double the fiber of conventional pasta.

1 28-ounce can diced tomatoes

1 tablespoon tomato paste

½ cup water

½ cup oat flour

⅓ cup grated Parmesan

½ teaspoon dried or freshly chopped oregano

¼ teaspoon freshly ground black pepper

1 egg

16 large shrimp, shelled, butterflied, tails removed (optional)

2 tablespoons olive oil, divided

1 head broccoli, cut into florets, stems discarded

8 ounces whole-wheat spaghetti, cooked according to the package instructions

Place the tomatoes and their juice, tomato paste, and water in a blender. Blend until smooth and set aside.

Spread the flour, Parmesan, oregano, and black pepper onto a sheet of waxed paper. Mix with your clean fingertips.

Place the egg in a shallow dish and whisk. Dip the shrimp into the egg and press into the flour mixture.

Heat a large skillet over high heat. Add half the olive oil. Add the shrimp and cook 4 to 5 minutes, turning occasionally, until the shrimp is lightly browned and cooked through. Transfer to a plate.

In the same skillet, warm the remaining olive oil over medium-high heat. Add the broccoli and cook about 1 minute, stirring occasionally, until the broccoli starts to brown. Reduce the heat to low and carefully add the tomato mixture. Simmer about 10 minutes, until the sauce reduces by half and the broccoli is tender. Add the pasta and toss to coat. Divide among four plates and top each with four shrimp.

447 CALORIES, 22 G PROTEIN, 12 G FAT (2 G SATURATED), 66 G CARBOHYDRATES, 9 G FIBER, 689 MG SODIUM

7 SUPERFOOD SNACKS TO SQUASH HUNGER

JUST LIKE DRESSING IN MATCHING OUTFITS WITH YOUR SISTER, snacking goes from a healthy behavior at kindergarten nap time to a habit many of us try to avoid in adulthood. But the problem isn't snacking itself; it's what we tend to snack on that gives rise to the idea that eating between meals is bad news for your weight. In truth, the right snacks can get you closer to your waist-whittling goal by ensuring that you never get famished between meals—and find yourself diving into pizza with the works.

The best time to snack: before you get too hungry. After each meal, your stomach's got a four- to five-hour capacity before it signals for more. Say you eat breakfast about 8 or 9 a.m., and lunch around 1 p.m. There's not much need for a midmorning snack, right? If you typically eat dinner at 6 or 7 p.m. or later, though, forgoing an afternoon fill-up can prompt you to choose a dinner that blows your diet; research from Georgia State University shows you're apt to eat more of it, too. But by having a little something left over in your stomach, you'll feel satisfied with a smaller meal.

The best snacks contain fiber-rich, unrefined carbohydrates, protein, and healthy fats to slow down digestion, boost your energy, and keep food off your brain. The recipes here do this automatically. Now, if only you could reinstate nap time, too!

LENTIL-PARMESAN HUMMUS

SERVES 8 • SUPERFOODS: Lentils, Olive Oil, Parmesan, Yogurt

This knockoff may look close to the chickpea original, but the creamy lentil-and-yogurt mixture makes for a skinnier dip, with less fat but more protein, fiber, and iron.

    1 cup dry brown lentils
    2 cups boiling water
    1/2 cup plain, low-fat Greek yogurt
    2 lemons, zested and juiced
    1/2 cup grated Parmesan
    2 tablespoons prepared tahini
    2 garlic cloves, minced
    1/4 cup warm water
    1 teaspoon extra-virgin olive oil
    1 teaspoon mild or hot chili powder
    2 carrots, peeled, cut into matchsticks
    4 stalks celery, cut into matchsticks
    1 red bell pepper, seeded, cut into matchsticks

Rinse the lentils under cold running water. In a small saucepan, bring 2 cups of water to a boil. Add the lentils and reduce the heat to low. Simmer 10 to 15 minutes, until the lentils are soft and the liquid has been absorbed.

Transfer the lentils to a food processor. Add the yogurt, lemon zest and juice, Parmesan, tahini, and garlic cloves. Process until a thick, chunky mixture forms. Add the water and process 10 to 15 seconds, until the mixture lightens in color and is smooth. Drizzle with the olive oil and sprinkle with chili powder.

Serve immediately with the crudités or store in an airtight container, refrigerated, for up to 5 days.

THE DISH (1/2 CUP) 167 CALORIES, 11 G PROTEIN, 5 G FAT (2 G SATURATED), 23 G CARBOHYDRATES, 10 G FIBER, 125 MG SODIUM

WASABI PEANUT POPCORN

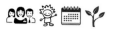

SERVES 8 • SUPERFOODS: Eggs, Peanuts, Popcorn

Popcorn may be the perfect whole-grain, low-calorie snack, but as with many other things that are good for you, it can be a little snoozy. This recipe wakes it up with a hint of sweetness and a little hit of heat for an anything-but-boring bite.

>   Olive oil cooking spray
>   6 cups air-popped popcorn
>   1 egg white
>   2 tablespoons wasabi paste
>   2 teaspoons brown rice syrup
> $1/2$ teaspoon salt
>   1 cup dry-roasted peanuts

Heat the oven to 200°F. Line a baking sheet with parchment paper or aluminum foil. Coat with cooking spray and spread out the popcorn on the paper. In a medium bowl, whisk the egg white, wasabi, brown rice syrup, and salt together until foamy. Add the peanuts and toss to coat.

Spoon the peanut mixture over the popcorn and transfer to the oven. Bake for 25 to 30 minutes, until the peanuts are golden. Remove and cool completely on the baking sheet.

Serve or store in an airtight container for up to a week.

 (3/4 CUP) 140 CALORIES, 6 G PROTEIN, 9 G FAT (1 G SATURATED), 11 G CARBOHYDRATES, 2 G FIBER, 155 MG SODIUM

HOMEMADE SWEET POTATO FRIES WITH BASIL DIPPING SAUCE

SERVES 4 • SUPERFOODS: Olive Oil, Parmesan, Sweet Potatoes

Sweet potato fries are flavorful enough to stand on their own as a side, but just as a cool handbag makes a simple outfit special, this supercharged dipping sauce transforms the fries into a solo snack star. The magnesium in the pumpkin seeds helps protect you against diabetes and belly-fattening metabolic syndrome, and their iron is energizing.

> 2 teaspoons cornstarch
> 2 large sweet potatoes, peeled, cut into
> $1/2$-inch wide wedges
> 2 teaspoons olive oil
> Olive oil cooking spray
> 2 tablespoons grated Parmesan
> $1/4$ teaspoon salt

Heat the oven to 400°F. Place the cornstarch in a large bowl. Add the sweet potatoes and toss well. The potatoes should be lightly coated and all the cornstarch used.

Heat two large, oven-safe skillets over medium-high heat. Add a teaspoon of olive oil to each and divide the fries between the skillets. Cook 2 to 3 minutes, turning occasionally, until the fries are slightly browned.

Slide the skillets into the oven, middle rack, and bake the fries 8 to 10 minutes, until the tops start to brown. Remove the skillets from the oven and flip the fries. Coat with a thin layer of cooking spray and return the skillets to the oven. Bake 15 to 20 minutes, until the fries are crisp but soft in the center. During the last 5 minutes of baking, remove the skillets from the oven and sprinkle the Parmesan over the top. Return to the oven.

Remove the fries from the oven and skillets and sprinkle with the salt. Serve immediately (see page 185 for a dipping sauce recipe).

 THE DISH (1 CUP FRIES, NO DIP) 151 CALORIES, 4 G PROTEIN, 3 G FAT (1 G SATURATED), 28 G CARBOHYDRATES, 4 G FIBER, 230 MG SODIUM

BASIL PUMPKIN SEED DIPPING SAUCE

SERVES 4 • SUPERFOODS: Olive Oil, Pumpkin Seeds, Yogurt

1 cup fresh basil leaves

$^1/_2$ cup plain low-fat Greek yogurt

8 teaspoons pumpkin seeds

4 teaspoons olive oil

2 garlic cloves

$^1/_2$ teaspoon salt

Place all ingredients in a mini chopper and blend until smooth. Serve with the fries.

 THE DISH (1 CUP FRIES PLUS DIP) 237 CALORIES, 5 G PROTEIN, 13 G FAT (2 G SATURATED), 29 G CARBOHY-DRATES, 3 G FIBER, 441 MG SODIUM

CHEF'S NOTE:

Want your snack even faster? Most frozen sweet potato fries are as healthy as those you'd make yourself, and sometimes it's worth paying for the convenience. But check the nutrition label and pass up any brands with trans fat (you'll sometimes see it hiding in the ingredients list as "partially hydrogenated oil").

APPLE ARTICHOKE QUESADILLA

SERVES 4 • SUPERFOODS: Apples, Artichokes, Olive Oil, Parmesan

Think of this snack as a mini, gourmet grilled cheese. Artichokes and apples deliver fiber, and sweet, sautéed onion adds fancy flavor. The cheese also sneaks in calcium, helping switch on your cells' fat-releasing power.

> 2 teaspoons olive oil
> 1 onion, cut into $^1/_8$-inch rings
> 1 tablespoon brown sugar
> 1 apple, cored, thinly sliced
> 1 teaspoon fresh thyme leaves, chopped
> 1 cup frozen or fresh artichoke hearts, defrosted and
>   chopped
> 4 whole-wheat or whole-grain tortillas (100 calories each)
> $^1/_2$ cup shredded part-skim mozzarella
> $^1/_4$ cup grated Parmesan, divided

Heat the oven to 400°F. Heat a small skillet over medium heat. Add the olive oil, onion, and brown sugar. Reduce the heat to low and cook 5 to 7 minutes, stirring occasionally, until the onion softens. Add the apple and thyme. Cook 3 to 4 minutes, stirring often, until the apple is soft. Stir in the artichokes.

Set out four tortillas on an ungreased baking sheet. Place a quarter of the mixture in the center of each tortilla. Top with 2 tablespoons of mozzarella and 1 tablespoon of Parmesan. Fold over and bake 2 to 3 minutes, until the tortillas are warm and the cheese has melted. Serve immediately.

243 CALORIES, 12 G PROTEIN, 8 G FAT (2 G SATURATED), 39 G CARBOHYDRATES, 11 G FIBER, 517 MG SODIUM

PEANUT BRITTLE

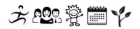

SERVES 20 • SUPERFOODS: Goji Berries, Peanuts, Popcorn

If you loved Cracker Jack as a kid, you'll find this sophisticated version just as crave-able. Peanuts hit the satiation trifecta of protein, healthy fats, and fiber, and popcorn adds whole grains. The two literally stick together to make this an easy snack to pop on the go.

> Olive oil cooking spray
> 2 cups air-popped popcorn
> $1/2$ cup white sugar
> $1/2$ cup brown rice syrup or golden cane syrup
> $1/4$ teaspoon salt
> $1/4$ cup water
> 2 tablespoons unsalted butter, softened
> 1 teaspoon baking soda
> 1 cup peanuts
> 2 tablespoons goji berries

Coat a large baking sheet with cooking spray. Spread the popcorn out over it and set aside.

Heat a heavy, 2-quart, saucepan over medium heat. Add the sugar, rice syrup, salt, and water and bring to a boil. Stir until sugar is dissolved.

If you have a candy thermometer, set it in place and continue cooking. Stir frequently until the temperature reaches 300°F. If you're not using a candy thermometer, stir until a small amount of the mixture dropped into very cold water separates into hard and brittle threads.

Remove from the heat. Stir in the butter and baking soda. (The mixture will thicken and foam.) Stir in the peanuts and goji berries. Immediately pour onto the baking sheet and press popcorn into the mixture. Allow to cool at least 1 hour at room temperature. Break the candy into twenty pieces. Store in an airtight container on the countertop up to 2 weeks.

 (1 PIECE) 96 CALORIES, 2 G PROTEIN, 5 G FAT (1 G SATURATED), 12 G CARBOHYDRATES, 0 G FIBER, 100 MG SODIUM

"EVERYTHING" KALE CHIPS

SERVES 4 • SUPERFOODS: Kale, Olive Oil, Parmesan, Pumpkin Seeds

These salty, crispy chips are addictive—but with only 125 calories per serving, double the fiber, and more than three times the protein of regular potato chips, you won't feel guilty about going back for more!

> 10 ounces kale, spines removed
>
> 2 teaspoons olive oil
>
> 2 tablespoons pumpkin seeds, chopped
>
> 1 tablespoon sesame seeds
>
> 2 teaspoons garlic powder
>
> 1/4 teaspoon freshly ground black pepper
>
> 1/4 teaspoon salt
>
> 1/4 cup grated Parmesan

Heat the oven to 400°F. Wash the kale under cool running water as you remove the spines. Dry the leaves well with a paper towel and tear into fist-size pieces. Place in a large bowl and add the olive oil.

Using your fingers, rub the oil over the kale leaves until they are well coated and shiny. Add the pumpkin seeds, sesame seeds, garlic powder, pepper, and salt. Toss to coat.

Split the kale between two ungreased baking sheets, spacing the pieces out into one layer on each sheet. Bake for 4 to 6 minutes, until they are crisp and brown at the edges. For the last minute of cooking, remove the baking sheets from the oven, sprinkle the kale with the Parmesan, and return to the oven.

Serve immediately, or cool completely before storing in an airtight container on the countertop for up to 4 days.

THE DISH (1 1/2 CUPS CHIPS) 125 CALORIES, 7 G PROTEIN, 8 G FAT (2 G SATURATED), 9 G CARBOHYDRATES, 2 G FIBER, 279 MG SODIUM

EDAMAME GUACAMOLE

SERVES 4 • SUPERFOODS: Avocado, Edamame

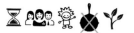

Meet the new hero of your next game-day buffet! With the addition of edamame, which is rich in fiber and choline to help block fat absorption, and soy protein to crank up your metabolism, this recipe crushes regular guac in taste and pound-peeling power.

1 cup frozen, shelled edamame, thawed

1 Hass avocado, cubed

1 large tomato, seeded and chopped

¼ cup cilantro leaves

¼ red onion, or 1 small shallot, minced (about ¼ cup)

½ small jalapeño, seeded, chopped

1 lime, zested and juiced

½ teaspoon salt

2 carrots, cut into matchsticks

1 large cucumber, thinly sliced

Place the edamame in a food processor and process until a chunky mixture forms. Transfer to a bowl and add the avocado, tomato, cilantro, onion, jalapeño, lime zest and juice, and salt. Stir to combine, mashing the avocado as you mix. Garnish with carrots and serve immediately with cucumber "chips."

 THE DISH (½ CUP GUAC, ½ CUP CUCUMBER, ½ CUP CARROTS) 152 CALORIES, 6 G PROTEIN, 8 G FAT (1 G SATURATED), 18 G CARBOHYDRATES, 7 G FIBER, 197 MG SODIUM

ROSEMARY PARMESAN POPCORN

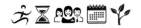

SERVES 4 • SUPERFOODS: Parmesan, Popcorn

Dressing up plain popcorn makes the low-calorie, high-fiber snack even more irresistible. Here, savory warm rosemary and Old Bay Seasoning (the latter is traditionally used in seafood recipes) deliver spicy flavor without much sodium.

> 1 tablespoon canola oil
> 1/4 cup popcorn kernels
> 1/2 cup grated Parmesan
> 2 tablespoons chopped rosemary
> 1/2 teaspoon Old Bay seasoning

Heat a large skillet over high heat for 30 seconds. Add the canola oil and popcorn. Cover immediately and shake the skillet as the kernels begin to pop. Cook 1 to 2 minutes, until the kernels stop popping. Remove from the heat, but keep in the skillet.

Sprinkle the Parmesan, rosemary, and Old Bay seasoning over the popcorn. Cover and rest 30 seconds to allow the Parmesan to crisp. Toss and serve immediately, or cool completely and store in an airtight container on the countertop for 1 week.

(1 HEAPING CUP) 114 CALORIES, 5 G PROTEIN, 7 G FAT (2 G SATURATED), 10 G CARBOHYDRATES, 2 G FIBER, 233 MG SODIUM

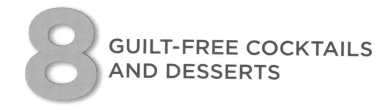

8 GUILT-FREE COCKTAILS AND DESSERTS

WHETHER IT'S A STRAPPY PAIR OF SANDALS THAT HAVE SOLD out or the perfect job you didn't get, nothing makes you want something more than being told you can't have it. That is precisely why this chapter is filled with decadent sweets, treats, and sips, that are just like your favorites. What's more, you'll enjoy portions you can actually savor at first sight, not itsy-bitsy bites you need a magnifying glass to appreciate.

The only difference between the goodies in this chapter and the desserts and cocktails you may be used to is that these only *taste* indulgent. Our magician of a chef perfected techniques and recipes that swap slim and satisfying ingredients—such as quinoa, yogurt, and fruit—for a percentage of the fattening ones. High calorie counts and grams of saturated fat *poof!* disappear, just like that, leaving behind sweet, rich flavors and the melty textures you love, plus a whole lot of healthy nutrients where empty calories once lived.

If you're following The *Drop 10 Diet* plan, you can spend your happy calories on anything you want, but we guarantee you'll get as much lip-smacking enjoyment out of these treats. Soon there will be a lot more room in your little black dress!

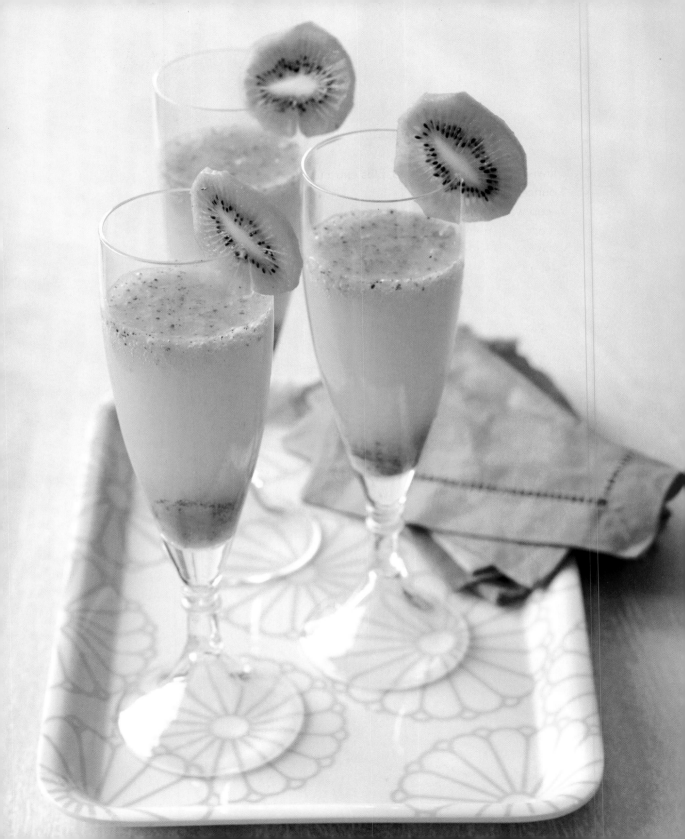

KIWI KIR ROYALE

SERVES 4 • SUPERFOOD: Kiwifruit

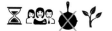

Here's to your health! This bubbly-with-benefits provides more than half your day's vitamin C, a nutrient that may help you burn fat, battle colds, and maybe fight cancer, too.

2 kiwis, peeled and quartered, plus extra for garnish
2 ounces triple sec
$\frac{1}{4}$ cup water
2 teaspoons powdered sugar
1 teaspoon vanilla extract
16 ounces champagne, chilled

In a blender, place the kiwis, triple sec, $\frac{1}{4}$ cup water, powdered sugar, and vanilla extract. Process until smooth. Strain.

Add $\frac{1}{4}$ cup of the kiwi juice into each of four champagne glasses; top each with 4 ounces of champagne and garnish with a slice of kiwifruit. Serve.

 168 CALORIES, 1 G PROTEIN, 0 G FAT (0 G SATURATED), 16 G CARBOHYDRATES, 1 G FIBER, 1 MG SODIUM

CHEF'S NOTE:
For the best flavor, ask your wine store clerk for a dry, crisp champagne or a prosecco with blossom notes.

PEANUTTY WHITE RUSSIAN

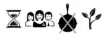

SERVES 4 • SUPERFOODS: Peanuts, Yogurt

You won't miss the cream in this sweet sip: The peanuts and Greek yogurt blend to create a silky, decadent-tasting mixer that skims 2 grams fat off your bottom line.

    $1/4$ cup plain low-fat Greek yogurt

    3 tablespoons dry-roasted unsalted peanuts

    2 teaspoons granulated sugar

    $1/2$ cup water

    6 ounces vodka

    4 ounces coffee liqueur

Place the yogurt, peanuts, and sugar in a food processor. Add the water and process until smooth. Add the vodka and liqueur and pulse until just combined, three or four times. Pour into four highball glasses filled with ice and serve immediately.

232 CALORIES, 3 G PROTEIN, 4 G FAT (1 G SATURATED), 24 G CARBOHYDRATES, 1 G FIBER, 8 MG SODIUM

POMARETTO SOUR

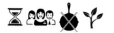

SERVES 4 • SUPERFOODS: Cherries, Pomegranates

If the mere mention of amaretto sours brings back memories from college, you're ready to graduate to this fresh update. Cherries, pomegranate juice, and almond extract replace sticky, nutritionally bankrupt sour mix and will help you turn back time to your senior-year size.

1 lemon, juiced
$1/4$ cup frozen or fresh black cherries
1 cup cold water
$1/2$ cup 100% pomegranate juice
4 ounces almond-flavored liqueur
$1/4$ teaspoon almond extract

Place the lemon, cherries, and 1 cup cold water in a mini chopper or blender and process until smooth. Strain and set aside.

Place the pomegranate juice, almond liqueur, and almond extract in a pitcher and stir. Add the strained lemon liquid. Fill four highball glasses with ice. Pour $1/2$ cup into each glass and serve immediately.

143 CALORIES, 0 G PROTEIN, 0 G FAT (0 G SATURATED), 10 G CARBOHYDRATES, 2 G FIBER, 4 MG SODIUM

BCG MARGARITA

SERVES 4 • SUPERFOODS: Blueberries, Cherries, Goji Berries

Thought the frozen cocktail was the forbidden fruit of dieting? Simply skip the sugary bottled mixes for this fresh-tasting concoction, which squeezes three sweet, fiber-rich superfoods and tequila into your glass for a slim 155 calories.

1 cup boiling water

1/4 cup goji berries

4 teaspoons granulated sugar

1 1/2 cups frozen blueberries

1 cup frozen cherries

4 ounces tequila

12 ice cubes

1 cup cold water

In a small saucepan, bring 1 cup of water to a boil. Stir in the goji berries and the sugar. Remove from the heat and let rest 15 minutes, until the gojis plump up and the sugar dissolves.

Transfer to a blender. Add the blueberries, cherries, tequila, ice cubes, and 1 cup cold water. Blend until smooth. Pour into four glasses and serve immediately.

 THE DISH 155 CALORIES, 1 G PROTEIN, 0 G FAT (0 G SATURATED), 22 G CARBOHYDRATES, 4 G FIBER, 22 MG SODIUM

CHEF'S NOTE:
To turn these fruity 'ritas into refreshing adult ice pops for a barbecue, blend all the ingredients, pour into molds, and freeze.

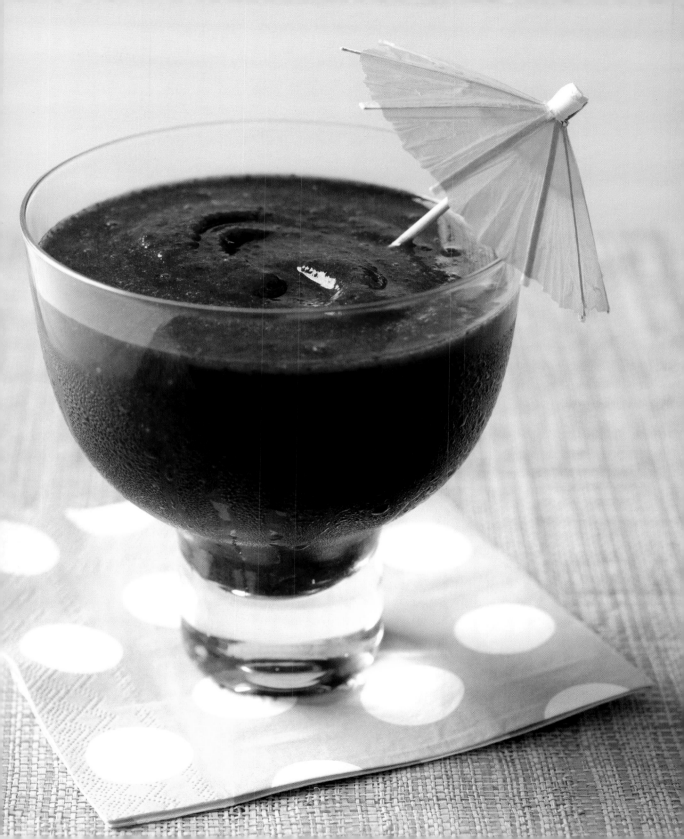

DRUNKEN MEXICAN COCOA

SERVES 4 • SUPERFOOD: Dark Chocolate

Happy calories, indeed! Sip on this cozy-with-a-kick hot chocolate after a cold day playing in the snow. Steamy and rich, with a touch of heat from cayenne pepper, it feeds your need for a warm-up and a sweet treat.

2 tablespoons unsweetened cocoa powder

2 tablespoons powdered sugar

2 tablespoons hot water

3 cups skim milk

1 teaspoon vanilla extract

$1/2$ teaspoon ground cinnamon

$1/8$–$1/4$ teaspoon cayenne pepper

4 ounces coffee-flavored liqueur

Place the cocoa powder and powdered sugar in a small bowl. Add 2 tablespoons of hot water and stir until a thick paste forms.

Place the milk in a small saucepan over medium heat. Cook 1 to 2 minutes, until the milk is hot, but doesn't boil. Whisk in the cocoa mixture along with the vanilla, cinnamon, and cayenne.

Set out four coffee mugs. Transfer $3/4$ cup of the hot chocolate mixture into each mug. Add an ounce of the liqueur, stir, and serve immediately.

 163 CALORIES, 7 G PROTEIN, 1 G FAT (0 G SATURATED), 34 G CARBOHYDRATES, 1 G FIBER, 80 MG SODIUM

CHEF'S NOTE:

Hold the liqueur to enjoy a satisfying hot drink for under 100 calories.

CHERRY BLOSSOM

SERVES 4 • SUPERFOODS: Cherries, Pomegranate

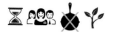

As gorgeous as they are light and refreshing, these fuchsia beauties let you embrace the retro cocktail craze while leaving extra calories firmly in the past.

$^{1}/_{2}$ cup frozen or fresh black cherries

1 cup 100% pomegranate juice

$^{1}/_{4}$ cup grenadine

6 ounces cherry brandy

8 ounces chilled, unflavored seltzer

Place the cherries, pomegranate juice, grenadine, and brandy in a blender. Blend and strain the liquid into a pitcher. Add the seltzer and stir to combine.

Set out four highball glasses and fill with ice cubes. Divide the liquid among the four glasses and serve immediately.

(1 CUP) 206 CALORIES, 0 G PROTEIN, 0 G FAT (0 G SATURATED), 24 G CARBOHYDRATES, 0 G FIBER, 8 MG SODIUM

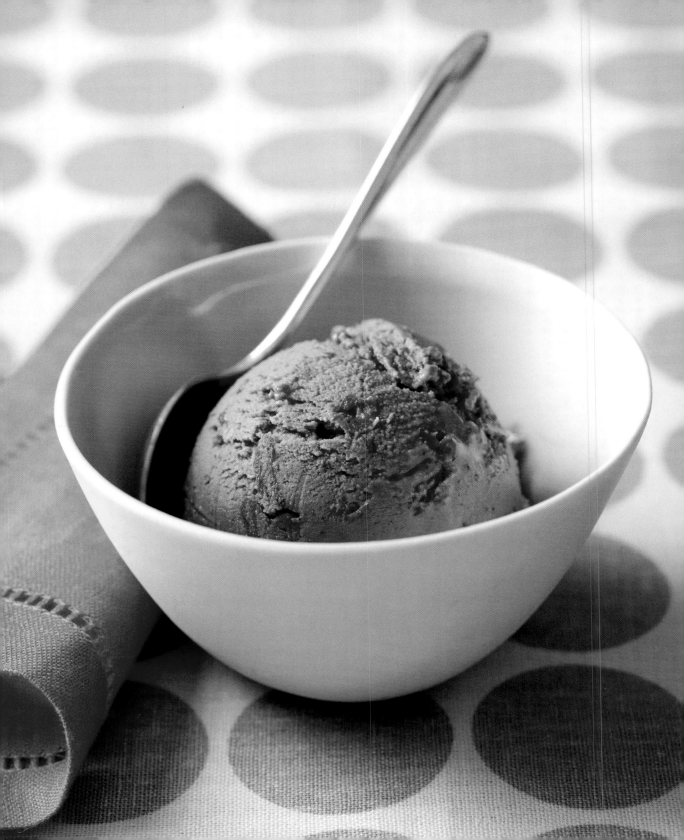

GOJI POMEGRANATE SHERBET

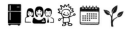

SERVES 8 • SUPERFOODS: Avocado, Cherries,
Goji Berries, Pomegranate, Yogurt

This cool scoop swaps out a lot of saturated fat for flab-resisting vitamin C and fiber. But don't worry, it's plenty creamy; even though you can't taste it, avocado brings a rich, luxurious texture to every bite.

> 1 cup frozen black cherries
> $^2/_3$ cup powdered sugar
> $^1/_2$ ripe Hass avocado (about $^1/_2$ cup)
> 2 cups plain, low-fat Greek yogurt
> 1 cup 100% pomegranate juice
> $^1/_2$ cup goji berries (2 ounces)

Place the cherries and powdered sugar in a food processor and blend. Add the avocado and process again until smooth.

Place the cherry mixture and the yogurt in a large bowl and whisk well. Gradually whisk in the pomegranate juice until smooth. Stir in the goji berries.

Freeze in an ice cream maker according to the manufacturer's instructions. Serve or store in an airtight container for up to 2 weeks.

THE DISH 176 CALORIES, 5 G PROTEIN, 2 G FAT (1 G SATURATED), 34 G CARBOHYDRATES, 2 G FIBER, 37 MG SODIUM

CHEF'S NOTE:
There's no need to defrost the cherries before blending.

SOFT CHOCOLATE CHIP COOKIE

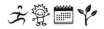

MAKES 40 cookies • SUPERFOODS: Dark Chocolate, Eggs, Oats, Olive Oil, Sweet Potatoes

There isn't one bit of butter in this recipe, but you'd never know it from the moist, gooey, and totally delicious results. The filling superfoods in it will leave you satisfied after just one—but at this calorie count, go ahead and enjoy seconds, sans guilt.

Olive oil cooking spray

1 ½ cups oat flour

1 cup "soft" white whole-wheat flour or whole-wheat pastry flour

1 teaspoon baking soda

¼ teaspoon baking powder

¼ teaspoon salt

½ cup packed light brown sugar

½ cup granulated sugar

⅓ cup light olive oil

1 cup finely grated sweet potato

2 eggs

2 tablespoons skim milk

2 teaspoons vanilla extract

1 cup 70% cacao chocolate chunks (break up a bar)

Heat the oven to 350°F. Coat three baking sheets with cooking spray or line with parchment paper. In a large bowl, place the flours, baking soda, baking powder, and salt and whisk to combine. Set aside.

In a separate large bowl, place the sugars and oil. Using an electric mixer on high speed, beat until a crumbly mixture forms. Reduce the speed to medium and beat in the grated sweet potato. Add the eggs, one at a time, and continue to beat until combined. Add the milk and vanilla extract and beat until the batter is smooth.

Reduce the speed to low and add the flour mixture and the chocolate chunks. Mix until just combined. Drop tablespoons of the dough onto the baking sheets, about 1 inch apart. Bake 7 to 9 minutes, until the centers of the cookies are firm to the touch.

Remove from the oven and transfer to a wire rack to cool.

(1 COOKIE) 86 CALORIES, 1 G PROTEIN, 4 G FAT (1 G SATURATED), 13 G CARBOHYDRATES, 1 G FIBER, 55 MG SODIUM

CHEF'S NOTE:
Cool cookies completely before storing. They'll stay fresh in an airtight container on the countertop for up to 5 days.

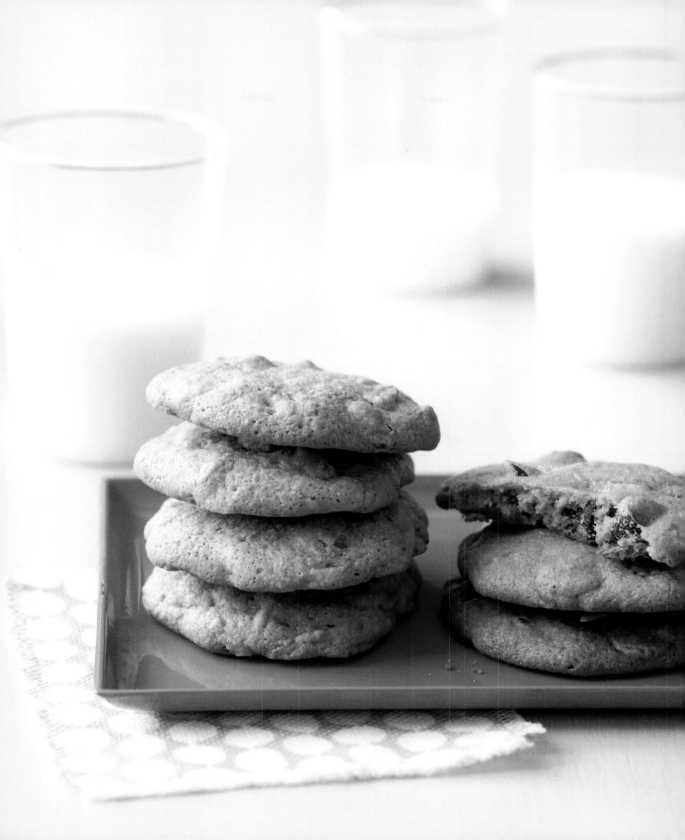

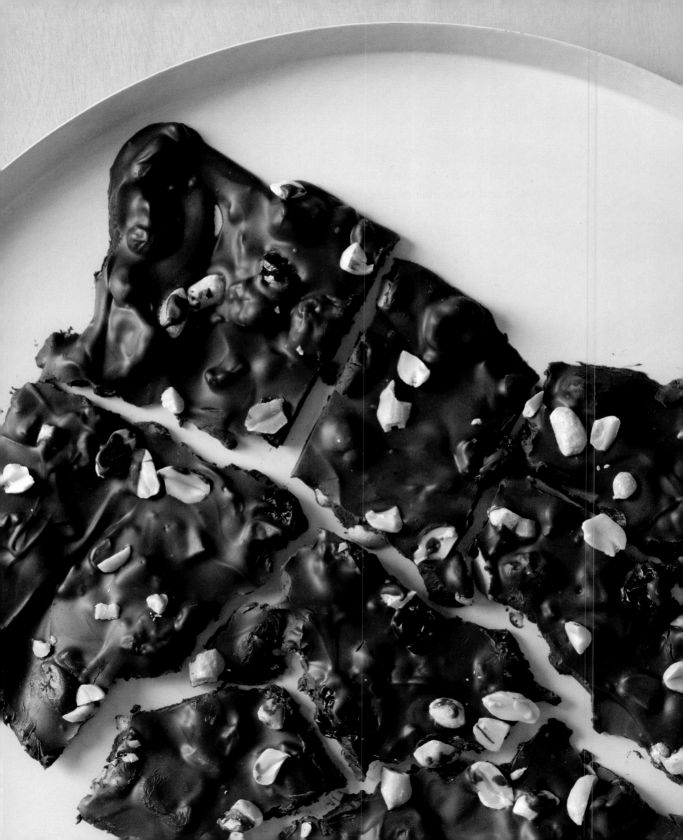

CHOCOLATE CHERRY NUT BARK

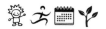

MAKES 9 servings • SUPERFOODS: Cherries, Dark Chocolate, Peanuts

Antioxidant powers, unite! The three-superfood team here may help save your heart, brain, and waistline in one miraculously chocolatey dessert.

8 ounces 70% cacao chocolate, 2 tablespoons finely
    grated and the remainder chopped
1/4 cup dried cherries, divided
1/4 cup chopped unsalted peanuts, divided

Line a 13 × 9-inch baking dish with parchment paper.

In a double boiler, heat the chopped chocolate over simmering water, stirring frequently, until almost melted. Turn off the heat, remove the insert from the pot, and stir the chocolate 1 minute. Let the chocolate cool, stirring occasionally, about 30 minutes.

Reheat the water in the pot over medium-low. Add the grated chocolate to the melted chocolate and return the insert to the pot. Stir constantly until the grated chocolate has melted. Turn off the heat, remove the insert, and stir in half the cherries and peanuts. Spread evenly onto the baking sheet. (Or to make clusters: Drop heaping tablespoons of the mixture onto the baking sheet, spaced about 1/2 inch apart.) Sprinkle the remaining cherries and peanuts over the top.

Cool on the countertop, uncovered, for 30 minutes. Cover with aluminum foil and refrigerate about 45 minutes, until the bark hardens (or clusters harden). Using a sharp knife, slice the chocolate block into uneven pieces for bark. Serve immediately, or store in an airtight container in the refrigerator for up to 2 weeks.

(2 PIECES OR CLUSTERS) 150 CALORIES, 2 G PROTEIN, 9 G FAT (5 G SATURATED), 20 G CARBO-HYDRATES, 2 G FIBER, 27 MG SODIUM

FROZEN BANANA YOGURT POPS WITH DARK CHOCOLATE DIP

MAKES 4 pops • SUPERFOODS: Cherries, Dark Chocolate, Goji Berries, Yogurt

Lick fat once and for all with these cool pops. Fruit bars are typically light on protein or fiber, but here you get both. The former revs your metabolism; the latter sends some of the fat packing before you absorb it.

1/4 cup (about 1 ounce) 70% cacao chocolate chunks
(break up a bar)
1/4 cup skim milk
1 cup plain, low-fat yogurt
1 banana, cut into chunks
1/2 cup powdered sugar
1/4 cup dried cherries
1/4 cup goji berries

Place the chocolate and the milk in a small saucepan. Stir continuously over low heat 1 to 2 minutes until the chocolate melts. Drizzle 1 tablespoon of the chocolate mixture into each of four ice pop molds. Set aside.

Place the yogurt, banana, and powdered sugar in a food processor or mini chopper and blend until smooth. Transfer to a bowl and stir in the dried cherries and goji berries. Divide the yogurt mixture among the four Popsicle molds and spoon on the remaining chocolate.

Freeze according to the manufacturer's instructions or for at least 2 hours before serving. Run the mold under hot water for 10 to 20 seconds to release and serve immediately.

THE DISH (1 POP) 218 CALORIES, 7 G PROTEIN, 4 G FAT (2 G SATURATED), 39 G CARBOHYDRATES, 2 G FIBER, 42 MG SODIUM

ORANGE-YOGURT CUPCAKES WITH PINK POMEGRANATE ICING

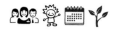

SERVES 12 • SUPERFOODS: Eggs, Oats, Olive Oil, Pomegranate, Yogurt

A cupcake can run about 230 calories—and that's before you ice it—but these festive treats let you have your cupcake and frosting for only 157. Yogurt replaces much of the oil, while keeping the crumb moist.

3/4 cup oat flour

6 tablespoons whole-wheat pastry flour

1/2 teaspoon baking powder

1/2 teaspoon baking soda

1/8 teaspoon salt

1/2 cup plain, low-fat Greek yogurt

1 orange, zested and juiced (2 tablespoons zest, 1/2 cup juice)

2 tablespoons light olive oil

3/4 cup granulated sugar

2 eggs

ICING:

1/4 cup plain, low-fat Greek yogurt

1/4 cup 100% pomegranate juice

2 ounces (1/4 cup) reduced-fat cream cheese, at room temperature

1/4 cup powdered sugar

1/2 cup pomegranate seeds (optional)

Heat the oven to 350°F. Line a twelve-cup muffin tin with cupcake papers.

In a large bowl, whisk together the flours, baking powder, soda, and salt. Set aside.

In a small bowl, place the yogurt, orange zest, and orange juice and stir to combine. (There will be lumps.) Set aside.

In a separate large bowl, place the olive oil and sugar. Using an electric mixer on high speed, beat until the oil incorporates into the sugar and a crumbly mixture forms. Reduce the speed to medium and add the eggs. Beat until the mixture is smooth and

(continued)

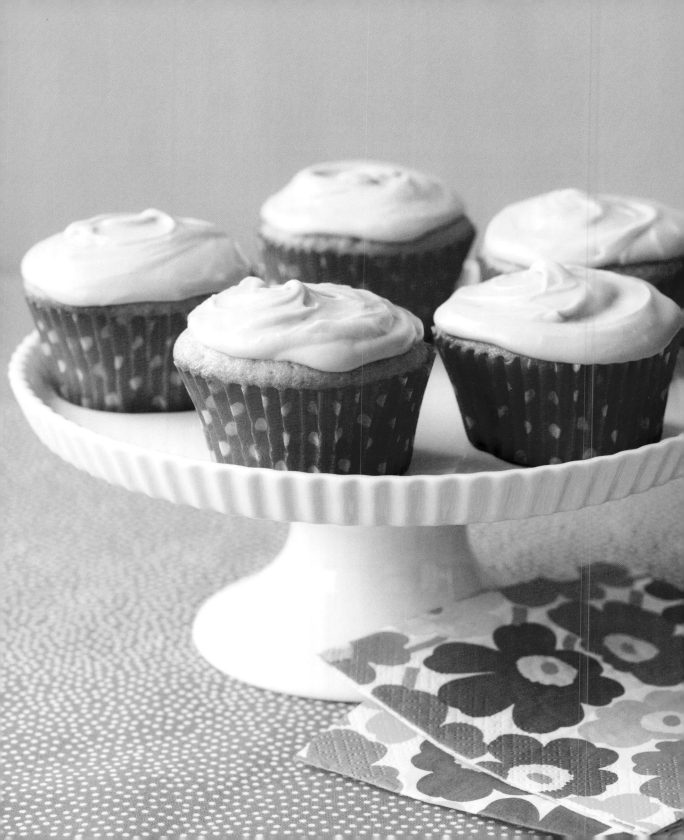

creamy. Reduce the speed to low and add half of the flour mixture to the bowl. Beat until most of the flour is incorporated. Add half the yogurt mixture and beat, scraping the sides, until the yogurt is just combined. Repeat with the rest of the flour mixture and the yogurt mixture. Pour the batter into the prepared muffin tins.

Bake for 15 to 20 minutes, until the cupcakes spring back when the tops are pressed or until a toothpick comes out clean. Remove the cupcakes from the muffin tin and cool completely on a wire rack.

PREPARE THE ICING:

In a medium bowl, place the yogurt. Gradually whisk in the pomegranate juice and set aside. In a separate large bowl, place the cream cheese and powdered sugar. Using a mixer on high speed, beat the ingredients 30 to 40 seconds, until very smooth. Reduce the speed to low and gradually add the yogurt mixture until icing is completely smooth.

Ice the cooled cupcakes and garnish with the pomegranate seeds, if desired (not shown). Serve immediately or chill, uncovered, until ready to serve (up to 8 hours).

 THE DISH (1 CUPCAKE) 157 CALORIES, 4 G PROTEIN, 5 G FAT (2 G SATURATED), 25 G CARBOHYDRATES, 1 G FIBER, 125 MG SODIUM

CHEF'S TIP:
If you'd rather not labor over a fresh pomegranate for a garnish, a thin slice of orange looks lovely, too.

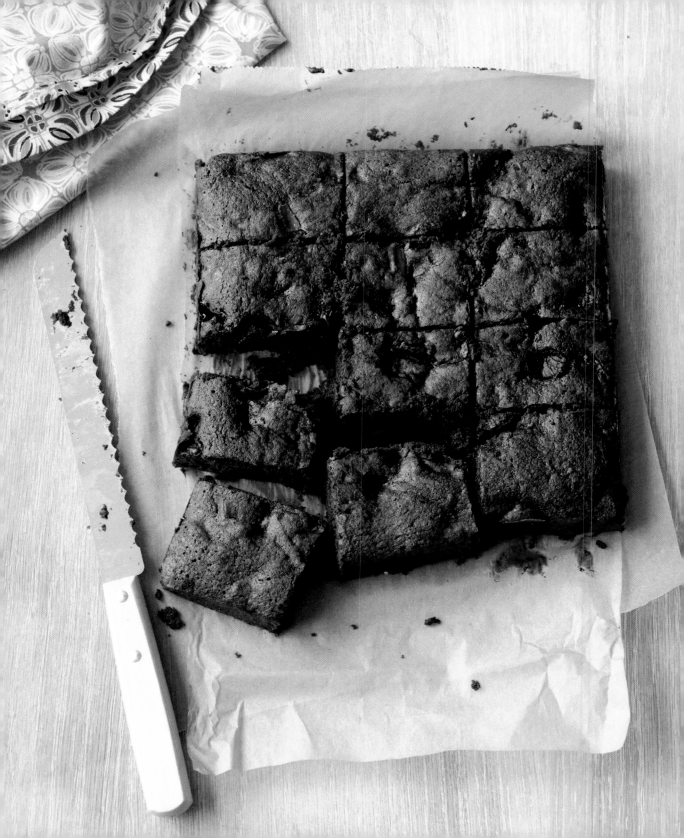

CHERRY CHOCOLATE BROWNIES

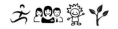

MAKES 12 brownies • SUPERFOODS: Cherries, Coffee, Dark Chocolate, Eggs, Oats

These fudgy, so-good squares are one tasty reason happy calories exist! Chewy cherries and whole-grain oat flour add fiber, while our chef managed to keep the calorie count at a manageable figure—to help you better manage your figure.

Olive oil cooking spray
1 cup oat flour
$1/4$ cup all-purpose flour
$2/3$ cup unsweetened cocoa powder
$1/2$ teaspoon baking powder
$1/8$ teaspoon salt
6 tablespoons unsalted butter, room temperature
1 cup granulated sugar
2 teaspoons finely ground coffee
2 eggs
2 tablespoons half-and-half
2 teaspoons vanilla extract
$1/2$ cup bittersweet chocolate chips
$1/2$ cup fresh or frozen cherries, chopped

Heat the oven to 350°F. Coat an 8 × 8-inch baking dish with cooking spray.

Place the flours, cocoa powder, baking powder, and salt in a large bowl. Whisk to combine well and set aside.

In a separate large bowl, place the butter, sugar, and coffee. Using an electric mixer, beat on high speed about 30 seconds, until a crumbly mixture forms. Add the eggs, one at a time, and beat on medium speed until a thick mocha-colored mixture forms. Add the half-and-half, the vanilla extract, and chocolate chips and beat on low speed until just incorporated.

Add the flour mixture and beat on low speed about 30 seconds, until a thick batter forms. Spoon the batter into the baking dish and press the cherries into the top.

Bake 25 to 30 minutes, until a cracked top forms and the edges are slightly firm to the touch, but the center is very soft. Cool in the pan for 30 minutes. Cut into twelve equal squares. Store in an airtight container for up to 1 week.

THE DISH (1 BROWNIE) 222 CALORIES, 4 G PROTEIN, 10 G FAT (6 G SATURATED), 32 G CARBOHYDRATES, 3 G FIBER, 89 MG SODIUM

CHEF'S NOTE:

These treats may seem underbaked when you take them out of the oven, but let them sit for 30 minutes—the "thirsty" oat flour will absorb the liquid and produce perfectly moist brownies.

COFFEE-CINNAMON PANNA COTTA

SERVES 4 • SUPERFOODS: Coffee, Yogurt

This Italian dessert—its name means "cream cooked"—is a blank canvas for flavor. Cinnamon and coffee taste luscious, and the latter helps improve your metabolism and sprinkles the sweet with stay-healthy antioxidants.

Nonstick cooking spray
$^1/_2$ cup skim milk, divided
1 tablespoon unflavored gelatin (1 packet)
1 teaspoon finely ground coffee
$^1/_2$ teaspoon vanilla extract
$^1/_2$ teaspoon ground cinnamon
$^2/_3$ cup powdered sugar
2 cups plain low-fat Greek yogurt
2 ripe bananas, thinly sliced

Coat individual 4-ounce molds or ramekins with nonstick cooking spray and set aside.

Place half the milk in a small saucepan. Sprinkle the gelatin over the surface of the milk; do not stir. Rest 15 minutes, until the gelatin creates a surface that resembles wrinkled fabric. Add the coffee, vanilla, and cinnamon and cook about 1 minute on low heat, until the gelatin and coffee dissolve. (Do not boil.) The mixture will be thick and speckled. Turn heat off and whisk in the remaining milk and the powdered sugar.

Place the yogurt in a medium bowl. Gradually whisk in the milk mixture until it is completely incorporated.

Pour into the prepared molds or ramekins and chill, covered, for 2 hours.

Coat a small skillet with cooking spray. Place over medium heat and add the bananas. Cook 1 to 2 minutes, turning once or twice, until the bananas brown.

When ready to serve, run a sharp knife around the inside edge of each ramekin. Place a small plate on top and turn over to release. Serve with the bananas on top.

THE DISH

216 CALORIES, 15 G PROTEIN, 2 G FAT (1 G SATURATED), 37 G CARBOHYDRATES, 2 G FIBER, 67 MG SODIUM

DOUBLE PEANUT BUTTER COOKIE

MAKES 40 cookies • SUPERFOODS: Eggs, Goji Berries, Oats, Peanuts, Quinoa

The monounsaturated fats in peanuts and peanut butter may prompt your genes to make you burn more fat and store less of it. They're also supremely satisfying, just like these rich treats.

Nonstick cooking spray
1 ½ cups oat flour
½ cup all-purpose flour
1 teaspoon baking soda
¼ teaspoon salt
1 cup cooked quinoa
1 cup packed light brown sugar

½ cup creamy peanut butter
2 eggs
2 teaspoons vanilla extract
½ cup dry-roasted, unsalted peanuts, chopped
¾ cup goji berries

Coat three baking sheets with cooking spray. In a large bowl, stir together the flours, baking soda, and salt until combined well. Set aside.

In a separate large bowl, place the quinoa, brown sugar, and peanut butter. With an electric mixer, beat on high speed until smooth and creamy. Add the egg and vanilla, and mix on medium speed about 1 minute, until the mixture lightens in color and is creamy.

Add the peanuts and goji berries, and stir with a wooden spoon. Add the flour mixture and stir until just combined. Cover and chill 1 hour.

Heat the oven to 325°F. Drop dough by heaping tablespoons onto the prepared sheets, spaced 1 ½ inches apart. Flatten slightly with the tines of a fork.

Bake the cookies 7 to 8 minutes, until the edges are firm but the centers are still soft to the touch. Let the cookies cool on the baking sheets about 5 minutes, until the centers begin to firm. Using a metal spatula, transfer the cookies to racks and cool completely. Store in an airtight container for up to 1 week.

(1 COOKIE) 79 CALORIES, 3 G PROTEIN, 3 G FAT (1 G SATURATED), 11 G CARBOHYDRATES, 1 G FIBER, 72 MG SODIUM

MINT CHOCOLATE CHIP FROZEN YOGURT

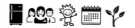

SERVES 6 • SUPERFOODS: Dark Chocolate, Pumpkin Seeds, Yogurt

This milky, frozen dessert is a true treat for your tummy: Fresh and indulgent tasting, it contains Greek yogurt to boost your calcium intake for maximum belly fat burn, plus probiotics to ward off stomach trouble.

2 tablespoons pumpkin seeds

1/2 cup fresh mint leaves

1/3 cup 70% cacao chocolate chunks (break up a bar)

2 cups plain, low-fat Greek yogurt

3/4 cup powdered sugar

1/2 cup skim milk

1/2 teaspoon mint extract

Place the pumpkin seeds in a clean coffee grinder and pulse until they are finely chopped. Transfer to a food processor. Add the mint leaves and chocolate chunks. Pulse ten to twelve times, until the mint and chocolate are roughly chopped. Add the yogurt, powdered sugar, skim milk, and mint extract. Pulse about five times, until a thick mixture forms.

Transfer to an airtight container and freeze at least 2 hours, or until firm. Defrost slightly 10 to 15 minutes before scooping and serving.

(1/2 CUP) 175 CALORIES, 9 G PROTEIN, 6 G FAT (3 G SATURATED), 23 G CARBOHYDRATES, 1 G FIBER, 32 MG SODIUM

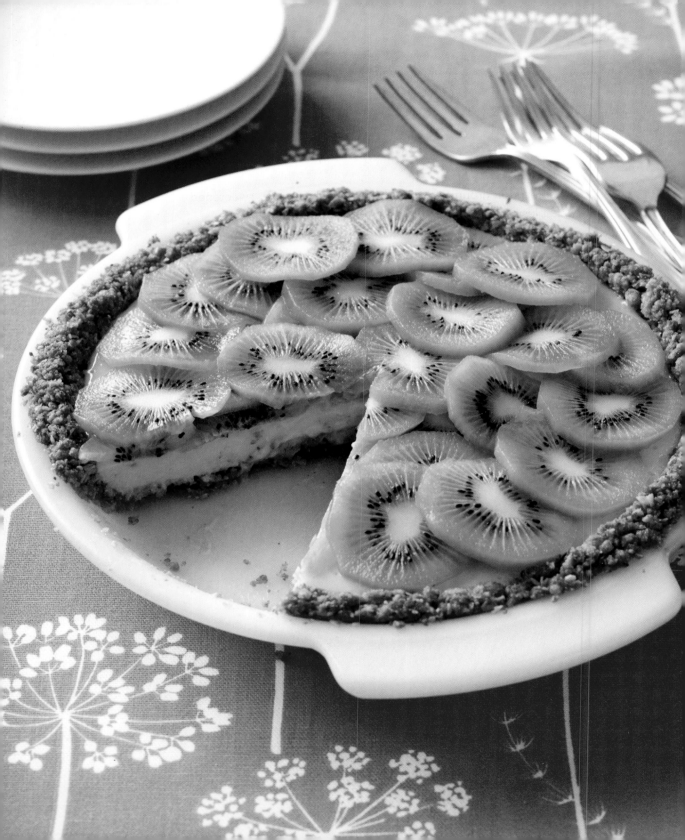

KIWI LIME PIE

SERVES 12 • SUPERFOODS: Eggs, Kiwifruit, Oats, Pumpkin Seeds

The tasty, tender graham cracker crust of this light pie subs pumpkin seeds and ground flax (both rich in unsaturated fats) for butter. You won't notice the difference, but your body will! These good-for-you fats readily burn fat off you.

1 tablespoon ground flax

2 tablespoons water

4 graham cracker sheets, broken in half

½ cup uncooked old-fashioned oats

2 tablespoons pumpkin seeds

1 14-ounce can sweetened condensed milk

5 egg yolks, beaten

4 teaspoons lime zest

½ cup fresh lime juice

4 kiwis, peeled, cut into thin slices

Heat the oven to 375°F. Place the flax and water in a small bowl and stir with a teaspoon. Set aside.

In a food processor, grind the graham crackers and oats into fine crumbs. Transfer to a separate bowl.

Using a clean coffee grinder, grind the pumpkin seeds. Add to the graham cracker mixture. Add the flax mixture and stir until a coarse meal forms. Press into the bottom and up the sides of an 8 × 8-inch pie plate.

In a large bowl, place the condensed milk, egg yolks, and lime zest and juice. Whisk well, until a thick, creamlike mixture forms. Pour over the unbaked graham crust and smooth the top with a rubber spatula.

Bake 12 to 15 minutes, until the edges are firm but the center still jiggles when you shake the pan. Remove from the oven and let cool 30 minutes. Decorate with kiwi slices. When the pie is fairly cool, cover with plastic wrap and chill for at least 1 hour, or up to 8 hours, before serving.

THE DISH (¹/₁₂ OF PIE) 219 CALORIES, 6 G PROTEIN, 7 G FAT (3 G SATURATED), 34 G CARBOHYDRATES, 1 G FIBER, 73 MG SODIUM

CHEF'S NOTE:
Add a spoonful of nonfat Greek yogurt to dress up your dessert even more (and sneak in another superfood!).

FRENCH APPLE TART

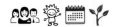

SERVES 8 • SUPERFOODS: Apples, Eggs, Oats, Pomegranate, Pumpkin Seeds, Yogurt

This stunner is pretty enough to appear in the window of any fancy bake shop, but even a novice can whip it up at home. The whole-grain oat flour adds slimming fiber and other nutrients that protect your heart.

1 cup oat flour

$^1/_2$ cup soft white whole-wheat flour or whole-wheat
    pastry flour

$^1/_8$ teaspoon baking powder

$^1/_4$ teaspoon salt

$^1/_4$ cup unsalted butter, room temperature

3 tablespoons sugar

1 egg

$^1/_2$ teaspoon vanilla extract

$^1/_4$ cup plain, low-fat Greek yogurt

Olive oil cooking spray

$^1/_4$ cup powdered sugar (for rolling out dough)

TOPPING:

1 medium apple, such as Golden Delicious, Pink Lady,
    or Gala, cored and thinly sliced

1 orange, zested and juiced (1 tablespoon zest,
    $^1/_2$ cup juice)

1 teaspoon ground cinnamon

Olive oil cooking spray

$^1/_2$ cup orange marmalade

$^1/_2$ cup pomegranate seeds

1 tablespoon pumpkin seeds, roughly chopped

In a large bowl, place the flours, baking powder, and salt. Whisk to combine and set aside. In a separate large bowl, place the butter and sugar. Beat with an electric mixer on

(continued on p. 220)

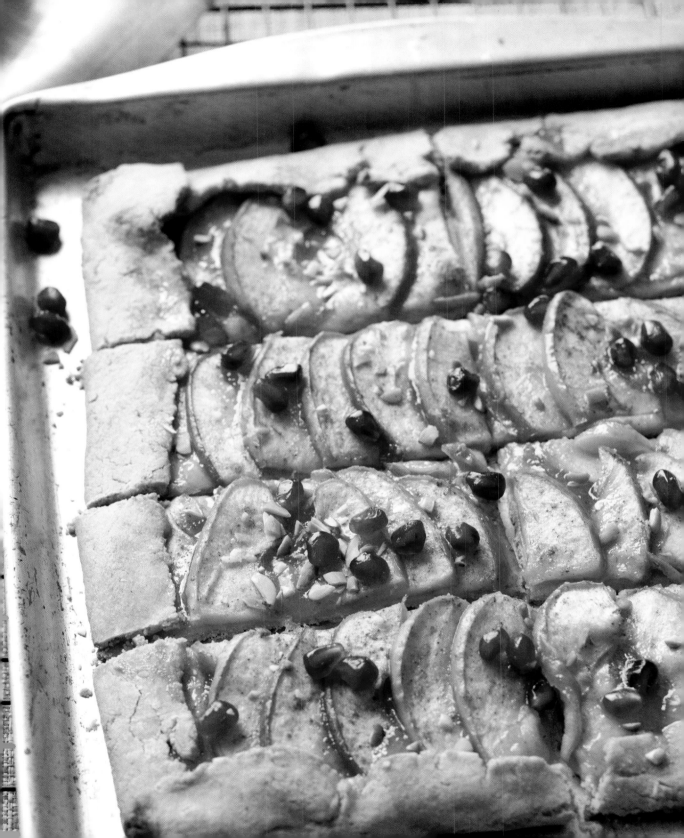

high speed until the mixture is pale yellow and light in texture. Reduce to medium speed and beat in the egg and vanilla until smooth.

Using a wooden spoon, stir in the yogurt. Add the flour mixture and stir until a soft, slightly sticky dough forms.

Coat a piece of aluminum foil or waxed paper with cooking spray and wrap the dough in it. Chill in the refrigerator for at least 1 hour before baking.

Heat the oven to 350°F.

PREPARE THE TOPPING:

In a medium bowl, place the apple, orange zest and juice, and cinnamon. Toss together and set aside.

ASSEMBLE THE TART:

Coat a large baking sheet with cooking spray. Place the dough on top. Sprinkle the powdered sugar over the dough and roll out into an 8 × 8-inch square. Using a rubber spatula, spread out the marmalade over the dough, leaving a 1-inch border around the edges.

Layer the apple over the marmalade in an overlapping pattern, so that only the edges of the dough remain visible. Drizzle with half of the juice from the bowl of apples. Coat the top with a thin layer of cooking spray and bake 20 to 25 minutes, until the apple is soft and the edges of the dough are golden and firm to the touch. Remove from the oven and drizzle with the remaining juice. Sprinkle with pomegranate and pumpkin seeds. Serve immediately or store in an airtight container for up to 3 days.

 ($\frac{1}{8}$ TART) 249 CALORIES, 5 G PROTEIN, 9 G FAT (4 G SATURATED), 42 G CARBOHYDRATES, 4 G FIBER, 100 MG SODIUM

ACKNOWLEDGMENTS

They say that too many cooks spoil the broth, but this book could never have happened without a dedicated crowd in and out of the kitchen. Each individual brought her own special sauce (so to speak) to the creative process, and I am eternally grateful for everyone's hard work and proud of the beautiful (and tasty!) result. In particular, I wish to thank:

The editorial experts:

Jennifer Iserloh, aka the Skinny Chef, for producing more than 100 delicious, healthy, and gorgeous recipes that can make the Drop 10 promise a reality for anyone who wants to lose weight without suffering for one second. Always cheerful and energetic, Jennifer truly understands how people like to eat and makes cooking nutritious meals fun as well as good for you.

Beth Janes, whose deep talent brings fresh energy to every word she writes. I dare you not to be motivated to make a positive change in your diet after reading the opening pages of Chapter 1. (Seriously, she made me try sardines!)

Marnie Cochran at Random House, who is the ultimate professional. Smart, funny, and unflappable, Marnie possesses the sort of experienced and decisive eye that is all too rare these days.

The creative pros:

Cynthia Hall Searight, *SELF*'s creative director, for lending her uniquely elegant vision to the planning and selection of the gorgeous photographs. The results here speak for themselves—you can't help but want to finish every last bite.

Linda Liang, *SELF*'s photo editor, who recruited the top team that prepared, styled, and photographed the food, and who produced the long and complicated shoot with seemingly effortless ease.

Photographer Kana Okada, for confirming our belief that healthy food can look every bit as good as it is for your body.

Food stylist Maggie Ruggiero and prop stylist Pam Morris, who together brought the dishes to appetizing life.

The research cops:

Pat Singer, *SELF*'s research director, for patiently and expertly directing the checking of the approximately 11 zillion facts in these pages. You can trust that the studies, science, recipe stats and more are as accurate as they can possibly be, thanks to the relentlessly diligent work of Pat and researchers Jacquelyn Simone, Marjorie Korn, Carlene Bauer, Trang Chuong, and Maura Corrigan. Thank you for dealing with all the inconvenient queries and late nights with grace and humor.

The master "chef":

Carla Rohlfing Levy, for her dedicated running of this team for the year it took for this brilliant idea to reach beautiful execution. She likes sardines now, too.

INDEX

Muffins (*cont.*)

    Devil's Food Cherry Chocolate Breakfast, 86–87

Mushroom Fontina Omelet, 68

Mushroom Turkey Meatballs with Angel Hair Pasta, 170

Mushrooms, 4, 21–22

    in breakfast recipes, 68

    in main meal recipes, 92–93, 98, 100, 108, 111, 116, 128, 132–133, 136–137, 149, 161–162, 166, 170, 174–175

N

Nachos

    Lentil Nachos with Cheese and Avocado, 116

NutritionData.Self.com, 10

O

Oat flour, 22, 33

Oatmeal, 22

    Cocoa Oatmeal, 62–63

Oats, 4, 22

    in breakfast recipes, 59, 63, 64, 65, 69, 81, 84–85, 86–87, 88–89, 90

    in dessert recipes, 202–203, 207–209, 210–212, 214, 217, 218–220

    in main meal recipes, 103, 104, 105, 131, 139–141, 143–144, 145–146, 147–148, 155–156, 166, 167–169, 170, 172, 178–179

Oils, 34

Oleic acid, 172

Olive oil, 4, 5, 22–23, 33, 69

    in breakfast recipes, 59, 64, 65, 66, 68, 76, 78, 86–87, 88–89

    in dessert recipes, 202–203, 207–209

    in main meal recipes, 92–93, 94–95, 97, 98, 101, 103, 104, 105, 106, 108, 111, 114–115, 116, 117, 118, 121, 122–123, 125–126, 127, 128, 131, 132–133, 136–137, 138, 139–141, 142, 143–144, 145–146, 147–148, 149, 150–151, 153, 154, 155–156, 157, 158–160, 161–162, 163, 165, 167–169, 170, 171, 173, 174–175, 178–179

    in snack recipes, 182, 184, 185, 186, 188

Omega 3 fatty acids, 6, 12, 19, 26–29, 106, 118, 136, 142, 173

Omelets

    Mushroom Fontina Omelet, 68

Onions

    Goji Lentil Salad with Caramelized Onions and Pineapple, 97

Orange Ginger Chicken with Pomegranate Quinoa, 145–146

Orange Yogurt Cupcakes with Pink Pomegranate Icing, 207–209

Oregano, 35, 36

Orzo, 28

P

Pan Roasted Shiitake Chicken with Apple Celery Root Puree, 161–162

Pancakes

    Chocolate Chunk and Cherry Pancakes, 65

Paprika, 35, 36

Paring knives, 39

Parmesan, 4, 5, 23, 31, 55

    in breakfast recipes, 66, 70, 76, 80, 84–85

    in main meal recipes, 98–99, 101, 104, 106,

Vinaigrette dressing, 34
Vinegar, 34–35
Vision health, 12, 15, 18, 19, 26, 28
Vitamin A, 123
Vitamin C, 15, 19, 20, 70, 80, 95, 108, 121, 123, 149, 153, 163, 173, 201
Vitamin D, 18, 19, 21, 26, 28, 29

W

Wansink, Brian, 37
Warm, Stuffed Caesar Mushrooms, 136–137
Wasabi Peanut Popcorn, 183
Water, 6, 13, 15, 21
Whole grain cereals, 33

Whole grain pasta, 4, 5, 28, 33, 50
    in main meal recipes, 94–95, 98, 106, 118, 138, 139–141, 150–151, 158–160, 170, 171, 174–175, 178–179
Whole wheat pastry flour, 33
Wild salmon, 4, 28–29, 50
    in breakfast recipes, 85
    in main meal recipes, 106–107, 139–141, 147–148, 155–156, 173, 176, 177
Wild Salmon and Pan Roasted Brussels Sprouts with Gojis, 173
Wild Salmon Ceviche with Mango and Avocado, 176
Wooden spoons, 42
Wusthof knives, 39

ABOUT THE AUTHOR

The editor in chief of *SELF* for more than ten years, LUCY DANZIGER is also the author of the *New York Times* bestseller *The Nine Rooms of Happiness*. Four years ago, she lost 25 pounds by eating more superfoods and has kept it off ever since. She is a regular guest on television shows, including *Today, The View,* and *Good Morning America*. Danziger lives in New York City with her husband and two children.

ABOUT THE TYPE

This book was set in Granjon, a modern recutting of a typeface produced under the direction of George W. Jones, who based Granjon's design upon the letter forms of Claude Garamond (1480–1561). The name was given to the typeface as a tribute to the typographic designer Robert Granjon.